DEFEAT DIABETES

MANAGEMENT, PREVENTION, AND REVERSAL

Publications International, Ltd.

Note: This publication is only intended to provide general information. The information is specifically not intended to be substitute for medical diagnosis or treatment by your physician or other healthcare professional. You should always consult your own physician or other healthcare professionals about any medical questions, diagnosis, or treatment. (Products vary among manufacturers. Please check labels carefully to confirm that the products you use are appropriate for your condition.)

The information obtained by you from this publication should not be relied upon for any personal, nutritional, or medical decision. You should consult an appropriate professional for specific advice tailored to your specific situation. PIL makes no representation or warranties, express or implied, with respect to your use of this information.

In no event shall PIL or its affiliates or advertisers be liable for any direct, indirect, punitive, incidental, special, or consequential damages, or any damages whatsoever including, without limitation, damages for personal injury, death, damage to property or loss of profits, arising out of or in any way connected with the use of any of the above-referenced information or otherwise arising out of use of this publication.

CONTENTS

INTRODUCTION

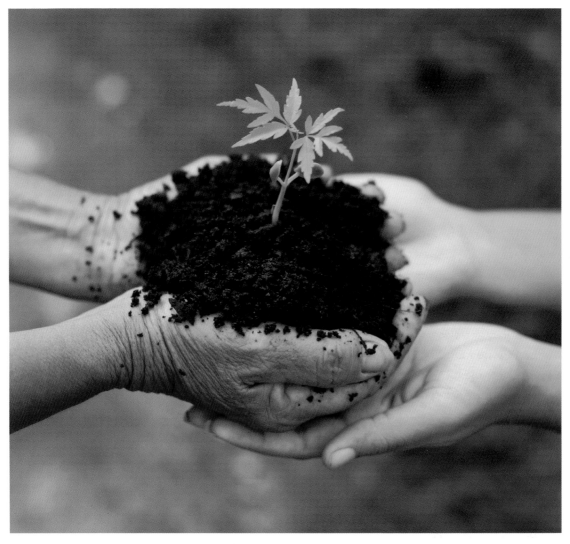

You don't have to be a prisoner of diabetes, living a life of deprivation, sitting there waiting for complications to develop. You can actively participate in your care, using the management tools at your disposal, to feel better and enjoy improved health and tighter diabetes control.

Taking Control

Managing diabetes can be a big, complex, ongoing job. If you've only recently received a diagnosis, the task of managing your disease can seem especially daunting. But *Defeat Diabetes* is here to help you tackle the task. You'll learn about how to assemble a care team, options for when and how to test your blood sugar, lifestyle changes that improve your health, how to prevent common diabetes complications, and your drug options and how diabetes medications work.

Finding Information

One tool at your disposal is information. Faced with a health problem, we sometimes want to bury our head in the sand. It's easier to avoid thinking about potential problems we may encounter, or lifestyle changes we may need to adopt. But the more you know, the better your chances at avoiding those potential problems. Knowing the facts about diabetes and being honest with yourself about your own health sets you up to manage your health in the most effective ways.

You'll find plenty of information in *Defeat Diabetes*. In the opening chapters, we cover the basics of the disease, explaining its causes, its variations, and its symptoms in terms a layperson can understand. You'll find information on the costs of unregulated high blood sugar, and the benefits you'll see when your blood sugar is under control. And you'll find ideas for how to assemble a care team that will help you manage the disease.

THREE KEYS TO TREATING, DELAYING, OR PREVENTING COMPLICATIONS

Education
- Learn as much as you can about diabetes.

Early detection
- Learn the signs and symptoms of potential problems.

Regular office visits
- Set up a schedule and stick to it!

In chapter 4, you'll learn about regulating your blood sugar, what supplies you'll need, and what your numbers should be.

Lifestyle Changes

Anyone who goes into a checkout line at the supermarket or looks at the array of magazines in a waiting room knows that there are a lot of suggestions out there for ways to lead a healthy lifestyle, from the newest trend diet to the latest exercise fad. Sifting out the suggestions you want to follow can prove difficult, and having diabetes only makes it more complicated.

However, the lifestyle changes you can make, including changes to your diet and exercise routine, are some of your most powerful tools in managing diabetes. Later in the book, you'll find tried-and-tested information about balancing your food intake, starting and maintaining an exercise program, and tips for controling your blood sugar.

Medication and Insulin

Not all people with diabetes take medication or insulin, but these can be powerful tools in your arsenal. While you'll need to discuss the specifics of your situation with your doctor and the rest of your care team, we provide an overview of the current available medications, including their strengths and potential side effects. We'll also look at the specifics of monitoring your blood sugar.

Preventing and Troubleshooting

Diabetes can come with a host of health complications. In the book's final chapters, you'll find material on preventing these complications, or handling them if they occur. Hypoglycemic episodes are one of the most common problems resulting from diabetes, and these are covered in chapter 9. In chapter 10, you'll find information on protecting your eyes, feet, and skin, so you can know what symptoms to watch out for, derailing any health issues as soon as they start.

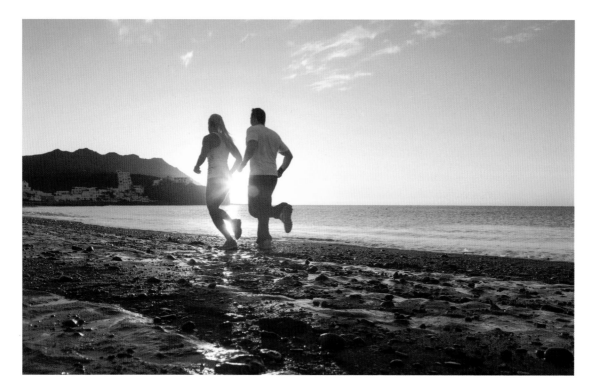

UNDERSTANDING THE PROBLEM

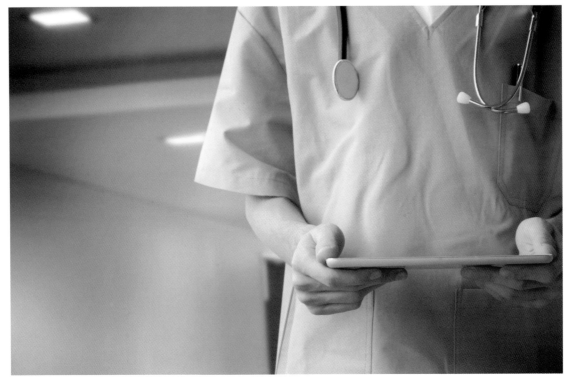

Diabetes is a problem with energy production. In medical terms, it's a metabolic disorder. If you have diabetes, your body can't efficiently use glucose, which is the body's main source of energy. It's not that you lack glucose. Unless you're fasting or on the All-Beef-and-Butter diet, you've got plenty of glucose in your system from the carbohydrates in the food you eat. The problem is getting the glucose into your cells, which need it to produce energy. The cells, for reasons we will explain, bar the glucose from entering. As a result, the glucose floats around in your bloodstream, slowly damaging everything in its path.

Fueling Up

Let's back up for a minute. To understand where the diabetic body goes awry, it will help to know how the body is supposed to process food and use it for energy. Humans can burn fat and protein as fuel, and in fact, muscles prefer to use fatty acids. But for the body as a whole, the preferred source of energy is carbohydrates, which it breaks down into a sugar called glucose. Glucose is the only fuel the brain can use.

When you eat a meal that contains carbohydrate, your body converts the carbohydrate into glucose during the digestion process. In a flash, the glucose enters the bloodstream—which is why glucose is referred to as *blood sugar*—and is quickly absorbed by the body's cells. Some of it is immediately used for energy, while the rest is placed into short-term storage—in the form of glycogen—primarily in the liver and muscle tissues. If you eat way more carbohydrate than you need for immediate energy and short-term reserves, your body will convert the glucose into fat.

If glucose could simply slip into your body's cells on its own, there would be no such thing as diabetes. However, glucose needs assistance from a hormone called insulin, which acts like a doorman, unlocking cells so that glucose can enter and be used as fuel.

The pancreas regulates insulin production. The pancreas actually produces a pair of hormones that regulate glucose levels in the blood. When the level of glucose in the blood begins to rise, the pancreas cranks out insulin to help get the glucose into the cells. When blood sugar levels drop too low, the pancreas produces glucagon, a hormone that travels to the liver with orders to convert some glycogen back into glucose and release it into the blood. With these two hormones, the pancreas helps you maintain a stable level of blood sugar.

You Just Can't Get Good Help

As mentioned earlier, people with diabetes don't lack for glucose—they have plenty. The problem is with the doormen. In people with type 1 diabetes, these gatekeepers never show up for work. In people with type 2 diabetes, the doormen arrive for duty but can't figure out how to unlock the gate. The result is the same in both cases: Glucose can't enter cells.

Type 1 Diabetes

If you have type 1 diabetes, the chances are pretty good that you have known it for a long time: Half of all people diagnosed with type 1 diabetes are younger than 20. In fact, type 1 diabetes used to be called juvenile-onset diabetes, back before doctors realized that the condition could actually strike people of any age. Another name sometimes used is insulin-dependent diabetes, since virtually all folks with type 1 require injections of the crucial hormone. Only about 5 to 10 percent of all people with diabetes have type 1, making it far less common than type 2 diabetes.

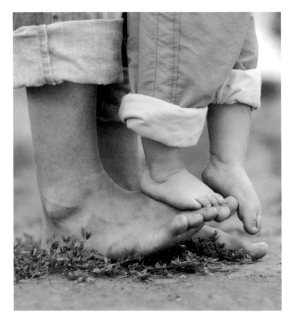

of many autoimmune diseases, which include rheumatoid arthritis, lupus, thyroiditis, and, yes, type 1 diabetes.

If you have type 1 diabetes, your immune system unleashed an assault on the cells in your pancreas that make insulin, known as beta cells. As your beta cells died off, your insulin production slowed down and may even have stopped. Without sufficient insulin to control the amount of glucose in your blood, your blood glucose levels began to rise, causing symptoms of diabetes. The symptoms likely included:

Type 1 diabetes begins with a glitch in the immune system, the body's defense against bacteria, viruses, and other unwanted invaders that roam around your body, trying to make you sick. The immune system is a complex network of vessels, fluids, white blood cells, and special proteins called antibodies that patrol your innards, looking for things that don't belong. When your immune system detects a germ or anything else that it doesn't recognize as belonging to the body, it fires off white blood cells and antibodies to engulf and destroy the intruder.

Unfortunately, in some people the immune system is guilty of friendly fire. It mistakes perfectly innocent and otherwise healthy body tissue for an enemy invader, attacking it with an onslaught of voracious immune cells. Depending on what part of the body your immune system attacks, the result can be one

- an unquenchable thirst. No matter how much liquid you guzzled, you still felt parched.

- a frequent need to urinate. Your bladder likely felt ready to burst whether or not you were gulping down fluids.

- increased hunger. You may have felt ravenous despite having recently eaten.

- sudden weight loss. Now you might be thinking, *Do you mean I get to eat like a pig and lose a few pounds at the same time? Sign me up!* Not so fast. Type 1 diabetes causes weight loss because your body is more or less devouring itself, which is not a good thing.

- unexplained fatigue. You probably felt drained no matter how much sleep and rest you got and how much food you consumed.

It's easy to see from these diverse symptoms just how important insulin is to the proper functioning of the human body. When glucose has no way of entering your cells, the sugary substance starts to build up in the blood. Your body has to pull water out of the blood (increasing thirst) so that it can get rid of the excess glucose in the urine (which explains the frequent trips to the restroom). Your cells are screaming for fuel. While they're waiting for more glucose, your cells switch to alternate sources of energy, so the body starts to run on fat. That's the reason you lose weight, but it's kind of like burning the furniture in the fireplace when you can't pay the heating bill. The combination of high blood glucose levels and dehydration makes you feel tired.

Burning fat all day instead of glucose isn't just inefficient; it can be life threatening if it goes on too long. As your body breaks down fat to use as energy, it produces leftover products called ketones. High levels of ketones are dangerous for the person with diabetes. Normally, these compounds pass harmlessly from your system into your urine to be excreted. But when carbohydrates are entirely removed from the diet—or when glucose can't get into cells, as in advanced diabetes—ketones build up to toxic levels. At first your breath has a weird odor, like fruit-flavored paint thinner. But soon you become confused, short of breath, and nauseous. You feel dehydrated and lose your lunch. If you don't get medical attention ASAP, you slip into a coma from which you may never awaken.

TYPES OF DIABETES

Type I diabetes

Type II diabetes

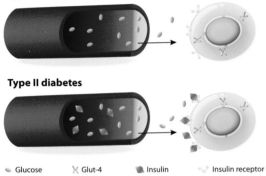

🌰 Glucose   ✕ Glut-4   🔲 Insulin   〵 Insulin receptor

Type 2 Diabetes

When your doctor uttered the words "You have type 2 diabetes," you were inducted into a fast-growing, nonexclusive club—a club no one wants to join. Some 90 to 95 percent of all people with diagnosed diabetes in the United States have type 2.

Like type 1 diabetes, this condition used to go by other names, including non-insulin-dependent diabetes and adult-onset diabetes. How times change. Now it's clear that both terms are misnomers. More than one-third of people with type 2 diabetes require insulin injections, so a person with type 2 diabetes may indeed be insulin dependent. And type 2 isn't limited to adults, either. While most people who develop type 2 diabetes are over 35, more and more kids are turning up in doctors' offices with classic type 2 diabetes, largely because more and more kids today are obese. As you read on, you'll learn why lugging around extra weight increases the risk for type 2 diabetes.

Unlike type 1 diabetes, type 2 diabetes is not an autoimmune disease, in which the body attacks its own cells. Type 2 typically begins with a phenomenon called insulin resistance, when cells throughout your body start to ignore insulin. The hormone comes knocking, but the doormen have trouble letting it in. The insulin may not be able to open the cell doors, or it may take reinforcements in the form of extra-large gushes of insulin before the cells will open up. In either case, glucose builds up in the blood.

Insulin resistance causes no symptoms. It's not as though you can feel or hear glucose molecules crashing into your resistant, tightly closed cells. However, insulin resistance often sets the stage for type 2 diabetes. Bottom line: If you have type 2 diabetes, you almost certainly have insulin resistance.

It usually takes insulin resistance months or years to progress to type 2 diabetes, when beta cells become progressively incapable of meeting the demand for insulin. At that point, insulin levels in the blood rise, too, as the beta cells keep cranking out the hormone in an attempt to coax open stubborn cells.

People often dismiss the signs and symptoms or blame them on some other health problem. A few indicators of type 2 diabetes overlap with those experienced by people with type 1, including:

- constant thirst
- frequent need to urinate
- increased hunger
- fatigue

However, type 2 diabetes often produces additional symptoms, such as:

- cuts that take a long time to heal
- frequent infections
- blurry eyesight
- tingling or numbness in the hands and feet
- erectile dysfunction

In all likelihood, your body began to experience insulin resistance long before you were diagnosed with type 2 diabetes, especially if you have any of the latter five symptoms. Excess glucose in the blood interferes with the work of white blood cells, which explains why cuts and sores take longer to heal. Meanwhile, germs snack on glucose, which makes them stronger, promoting more infections. Long-term exposure to glucose damages nerves, too, which explains many other symptoms of type 2 diabetes.

While you may be able to live with these problems, they should serve as a clear warning that your out-of-control blood sugar is slowly trashing your body like a rowdy rock band wrecks a hotel room. Left untreated, type 2 diabetes—or any type of diabetes, for that matter—can lead to medical catastrophe.

Gestational Diabetes

You're stuck wearing maternity clothes. You miss having a glass of wine with dinner. You can't see your feet when you stand up. And now you find out that your pregnancy is causing diabetes? Talk about frustrating! Gestational diabetes may affect anywhere from 2 to 18 percent of pregnancies. The condition usually doesn't arise until after 20 weeks of pregnancy. And while any pregnant woman can develop gestational diabetes, it's more common if you:

- are older than 25
- have a parent or sibling with diabetes
- are African American, American Indian, Asian American, Hispanic American, or Pacific Islander
- are overweight
- developed gestational diabetes during a previous pregnancy or have given birth to an infant who weighed more than nine pounds
- have ever been told by a doctor that you have prediabetes, impaired glucose tolerance, or impaired fasting glucose

So what's the harm in having high blood sugar for a few months? For starters, women with gestational diabetes often develop high blood pressure (referred to as pre-eclampsia), which brings its own risks for both mother and baby. What's more, they frequently give birth to very large babies who weigh more than nine pounds. Not only do fat babies often require a caesarean-section delivery, they're also more likely to be fat children and to develop diabetes by their teen years or young adulthood (because of their genetic inheritance, not the intrauterine environment).

The news about gestational diabetes isn't all bad. After all, there's a reliable cure for the problem: having your baby, after which most women's blood sugar levels return to nomal.

However, the condition lingers in a small number of women, who are then diagnosed with either type 1 or type 2 diabetes. Regardless, if you have gestational diabetes once, the odds are two out of three that you'll develop it again with a subsequent pregnancy. More concerning, women who have gestational diabetes stand a 20 to 50 percent risk of developing type 2 diabetes within a decade.

OTHER TYPES OF DIABETES

Type 1, type 2, and gestational diabetes are the main types of the disease, but they're not the only ones. The following are other diabetes permutations.

"Double Diabetes"

Although it's not a term you will find in most medical textbooks, many doctors today say they are treating a growing number of type 1 diabetes patients who have also developed insulin resistance, the classic symptom of type 2 diabetes. Some doctors are treating these hybrid patients with drugs that make their bodies more sensitive to insulin. The term "double diabetes" may also be used to describe a person with type 2 diabetes who develops antibodies that destroy pancreatic beta cells (the ones that produce insulin); in most cases, these patients will require insulin injections. Just to make matters more confusing, double diabetes is sometimes called type 3 diabetes.

Prediabetes

Think of it as the diabetic gray zone. You have insulin resistance, but it's not high enough for

BY THE NUMBERS

Here are some quick facts about diabetes, according to the latest available National Diabetes Fact Sheet:

- 29.1 million Americans—9.3 percent of the population—have diabetes (diagnosed and undiagnosed cases).

- 8.1 million Americans have diabetes but don't know it.

- 12.3 percent of Americans aged 20 years and older have diabetes.

- 1.7 million Americans aged 20 years and older are diagnosed with diabetes each year.

you to be diagnosed with type 2 diabetes. (We'll explain the values doctors use to measure blood sugar later.) It has been estimated that about 86 million Americans aged 20 years and older have prediabetes. Most people who have the condition develop full-blown type 2 diabetes within 10 years. However, making certain changes, such as losing weight, can delay or even prevent that from happening.

Latent Autoimmune Diabetes of Adulthood (LADA)

LADA is also known as slow-onset type 1 diabetes. Call them late bloomers: About 5 to 10 percent of people with diabetes are adults who develop the type 1 variety of the condition, which is typically first diagnosed in children and teens. Doctors often mistake the condition for plain old type 2 diabetes, basing their diagnosis solely on a patient's age and high blood sugar. But people with LADA don't have insulin resistance and aren't necessarily overweight. Those are important distinctions, since they influence which treatments work for LADA.

Maturity-Onset Diabetes of the Young (MODY)

MODY is something like the flipside of LADA. It usually turns up in teens and young adults, although it may be found in children as well as older adults. Because patients tend to be youngish and slender, doctors often misdiagnose the condition as type 1 diabetes. MODY, however, is a genetic disorder that interferes with insulin production. And unlike people with type 2 diabetes, those with MODY don't have insulin resistance. Again, getting the right diagnosis is critical in order to choose the proper treatment approach for MODY.

Secondary Diabetes

Certain diseases and drug therapies pack a diabetic double whammy by making people more vulnerable to blood sugar problems,

INSULIN AND YOUR HEART

Too much of a good thing can make you sick. That rule applies to insulin in a big way. While you need insulin to survive, sending gushers of the hormone into your blood can eventually damage arteries, which makes insulin resistance a cause of heart disease.

Insulin resistance is one part of a spectrum of conditions that make up the medical threat originally known as Syndrome X, but now more commonly called metabolic syndrome or insulin resistance syndrome. The National Cholesterol Education Program defines metabolic syndrome as the presence of any three of the following conditions:

- Excess weight around the waist (a waist measurement of more than 40 inches for men and more than 35 inches for women)
- High levels of blood fats called triglycerides (150 mg/dl or higher)
- Low levels of HDL ("good") cholesterol (below 40 mg/dl for men and below 50 mg/dl for women)
- High blood pressure (130/85 or higher)
- High fasting blood glucose levels (110 mg/dl or higher)

Other medical organizations use slightly different criteria for defining metabolic syndrome. And some doctors don't think metabolic syndrome exists at all, since it has no single cause. In addition to the cluster of factors mentioned above, other culprits include high levels of inflammation in the blood vessels and disorders that damage the endothelium, or lining of blood vessels.

either by directly interfering with insulin or by producing physical changes that increase insulin resistance (such as weight gain) and can lead to diabetes. When another identifiable medical problem or medication precipitates the development of diabetes, it is called secondary diabetes. A brief list of conditions that may cause secondary diabetes includes depression, HIV, pancreatitis, certain hormonal disorders (such as Cushing's syndrome and hyperthyroidism), and some genetic disorders (such as cystic fibrosis). Drugs linked to secondary diabetes include diuretics and other drugs used to treat high blood pressure, steroid hormones, certain asthma medications, antidepressants, anticonvulsants, and some forms of cancer chemotherapy, among others.

WHAT CAUSES DIABETES?

Scientists have pinpointed a number of genes that seem to be involved in creating your body's blood sugar problems. Yet they also know that one or more triggers in the environment are probably necessary, too. But what are those potential triggers? And how do they keep insulin from doing its job? Researchers are still sorting out these questions, but here's a look at what they know so far.

Type 1 Diabetes

If you have type 1 diabetes, there's a good chance one of your parents passed along to you an abnormal gene or cluster of genes that puts you at greater-than-average risk for developing the condition. (For those of you who were busy dozing or passing notes during high school biology class, everyone inherits a blend of genes from both parents that not only determines what you look like but also greatly influences your health.)

Being born with these genes doesn't guarantee that you will develop type 1 diabetes, however. These inherited genes only make you *susceptible* to developing diabetes. Something else has to trigger changes in your body to create your blood sugar problem. But what? Scientists aren't sure, but they have a short list of suspects. According to one theory, a virus or some environmental toxin worms its way into the body and confuses the immune system because it resembles proteins found on beta cells. The immune system tends to shoot first and ask questions later, so it destroys anything that looks like it could be a threat— including insulin-producing beta cells in the pancreas. Type 1 diabetes occurs more often in people who have had a viral illness, as this can trigger the onset of type 1 diabetes in a susceptible individual.

Other scientists have speculated that switching a baby from breast milk to cow's milk too early is the culprit. However, the dairy-diabetes connection remains controversial. In fact, in 2003 a pair of studies in the *Journal of the American Medical Association* found no connection between consuming cow's milk and diabetes. Some causes are more clear-cut. For example, certain prescription medications can trigger type 1 diabetes.

Type 2 Diabetes

If you have type 2 diabetes, you may have begun to regret every can of cola and candy bar you ever consumed. After all, if high blood glucose is your problem, didn't gobbling and guzzling all that sugar cause you to develop diabetes?

The precise answer to that question is "Not exactly," though having a sweet tooth probably didn't help matters. Despite the common misconception, consuming sugary foods doesn't cause diabetes. However, eating too much of most any kind of food—whether it's bonbons or bacon cheeseburgers—can make you gain weight. And getting fat worsens insulin resistance, the problem that's at the core of type 2 diabetes.

Insulin resistance is the medical term for the concept described earlier: Cells throughout your body have begun to ignore insulin, so your pancreas keeps cranking out more of the hormone to move glucose past those stubborn cell membranes.

What causes insulin resistance? Typically, it's a combination of genetics (heredity) and lifestyle. Family history plays a major role. Having close relatives with type 2 diabetes greatly increases your risk of the disease. Certain ethnic groups, including American Indians, African Americans, Hispanic Americans, Asian Americans, and Pacific Islanders are also at high risk. The aging process plays a role, too. The older we get, the more insulin resistant we tend to become, so the risk of developing type 2 diabetes increases with age.

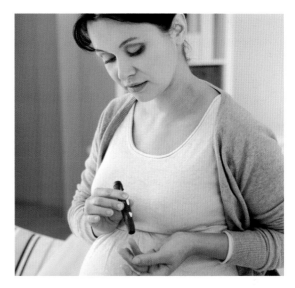

Women who have a condition called polycystic ovary syndrome (PCOS) often become insulin resistant due to the overproduction of certain hormones that work against insulin's action.

Likewise, several hormones produced during pregnancy fight against insulin's action and can cause insulin resistance. And as noted earlier, women who develop gestational diabetes during pregnancy or have given birth to a large or heavy baby are at increased risk of developing type 2 diabetes as they get older.

Stressful circumstances, such as illness, injury, surgery, or daily emotional turmoil, can cause significant insulin resistance. This is due to the production of stress hormones. These hormones normally prompt the surge of energy needed for a "fight or flight" response in stressful situations. Unfortunately for people

prone to diabetes, the stress hormones trigger this energy burst by stimulating the liver to release extra sugar into the bloodstream and by causing insulin resistance.

A number of medications can also produce insulin resistance, most notably, anti-inflammatory steroid drugs such as cortisone and prednisone. These types of drugs create a state of insulin resistance throughout the body.

A lack of physical activity can cause insulin resistance in many people. The muscles are one of the primary consumers of sugar for energy. When muscle function is limited to little more than getting up to find the remote or to head to the fridge, muscles start to lose their sensitivity to insulin. Even in people who are usually very active, a couple of days without much activity will result in some degree of insulin resistance.

Last but certainly not least, insulin resistance

increases with body size. But let's get the terminology straight. We're not talking about being big and muscular. We're talking about having too much body fat, particularly around the midsection. Obesity is far and away the number one risk factor for type 2 diabetes. We don't know exactly how body fat gets in the way of insulin. But we do know that fat cells secrete a hormone that limits insulin's ability to promote sugar uptake by the body's cells. The larger your fat cells, the more of this hormone you produce, and the greater your degree of insulin resistance. In fact, gaining as little as ten pounds over a 15-year period can double your level of insulin resistance.

Still, if some 86 million Americans have insulin resistance, why have less than half of them developed type 2 diabetes? Why the discrepancy? The reason is this: When insulin resistance occurs, the pancreas needs to produce more insulin to keep blood sugar levels in a normal range. In most cases, the pancreas can produce enough extra insulin to keep blood sugar levels out of the diabetic range, even though the insulin is not working as well as it should. This is the prediabetes phase.

But not everyone's pancreas has this capacity. Each person's pancreas can only crank up insulin production so much. Once the degree of insulin resistance is too much for the pancreas to overcome, blood sugar levels are going to rise above normal. In other words, a body must have both insulin resistance *and* a limit to its ability to secrete extra insulin in order for type 2 diabetes to occur.

Imagine you're an air conditioner trying to keep the house cool on a hot summer day. If you're one of those high-powered units that can crank out a bazillion BTUs, you'll have no problem keeping the house cool. But if you're just an inexpensive window unit, you're probably not going to be able to blow enough cold air to keep the entire house cool on a really hot day. In this example, the heat and humidity are like insulin resistance: They present a challenge to our comfort and well-being. The air conditioner is like the pancreas: An efficient system can overcome any challenge, but a less-resilient system can't. When a sluggish pancreas combines with major insulin resistance, the result is going to be type 2 diabetes.

Fortunately, at this early stage of type 2 diabetes, blood sugar control can often be achieved through exercise and a healthy diet. Physical activity helps the body overcome insulin resistance. Consuming fewer carbohydrates helps to limit the amount of sugar entering the bloodstream at any one time. And the combination of exercise and reduced food intake produces weight loss, which also improves insulin sensitivity. Sometimes at this stage, however, oral medications may also be needed to help the pancreas (or to help insulin) work more effectively. Combined with the lifestyle adjustments, they may be sufficient to rein in blood sugar levels, at least for a while.

However, type 2 diabetes is a progressive illness. When diabetes has been present for

NO COINCIDENCE

In a Gallup-Healthways survey conducted in 2012, six of the ten states with the highest obesity rates were also among the ten states with the highest rates of diabetes. Those states were (in alphabetical order):

Alabama, Kentucky, Louisiana, Mississippi, Tennessee, and West Virginia.

percent of the people with type 2 diabetes take insulin injections, sometimes several times each day. Does this mean they now have type 1 diabetes? No, it does not. Remember, the type of diabetes is defined by what *caused* it, not how it is treated. Type 1 diabetes occurs when the body's own immune system destroys the part of the pancreas that makes insulin. Type 2 diabetes is caused by insulin resistance (usually due to obesity and family history/ethnicity), followed by insufficient insulin production (as the pancreas fails to keep up with the increased demand), followed by a gradual breakdown of the pancreas (due to constant overwork and glucose toxicity).

How Does My Doctor Know I Have Diabetes?

Your blood sugar gives you away, of course. Doctors do look for other clues when considering a diagnosis of diabetes—outward symptoms, for example, or the presence of risk factors, such as overweight or a family history of the disease. But a firm diagnosis of diabetes isn't made until the blood is tested.

a number of years, insulin resistance tends to grow worse, and the pancreas struggles to keep up with the huge demand for insulin. Then a new problem typically sets in. Just like an air conditioner that is forced to run full blast every minute of every day, the pancreas starts to break down. The breakdown of the pancreas has two causes—overwork and a condition known as glucose toxicity. We can all understand the overwork part: Force those poor little pancreatic cells into relentless labor, and many of them are going to bite the dust. But glucose toxicity is a bit more complex.

Glucose is a good thing in the right amounts. But elevations in blood sugar levels can actually damage the pancreas, further reducing its ability to produce insulin. So over time, because of the constant battle against insulin resistance, the pancreas starts to make less and less insulin. This is why the treatment for type 2 diabetes usually must become more aggressive over time. It is why roughly 40

If a patient walks in complaining that he or she is unusually thirsty and always dashing for the restroom, for instance, a physician may suspect diabetes, especially the type 1 variety. But the diagnosis can't be confirmed until the blood sugar level is tested. For a patient exhibiting symptoms that are common with diabetes, a doctor may order a *random blood glucose (RBG)* test. This test can be performed at any time and doesn't require preparation. A result that shows a blood sugar level more than 200 milligrams per deciliter (mg/dl) suggests diabetes is present. Since prediabetes and the early stages of type 2 diabetes often don't cause outward symptoms, a doctor may order a blood test called an *HbA1c,* often shortened to *A1c,* to check for diabetes in a patient who is over age 45 (the risk of type 2 diabetes increases with age), is overweight, or has any other risk factor for the disease. At one time, A1c testing was used only as a method for evaluating diabetes management. But in 2009, an international committee of diabetes experts determined that the test could also be used in most cases for diagnosing prediabetes and type 2 diabetes. Like an RBG test, an A1c test can be performed at any time of day and doesn't require fasting beforehand. The A1c results reflect a patient's average blood glucose level over the previous two to three months. An A1c of 5.7 to 6.4 indicates prediabetes; a level of 6.5 or above means the patient has diabetes.

Another option for diagnosing prediabetes and diabetes is a *fasting plasma glucose (FPG)* test. This test is more definitive than an RBG test and is often included in the routine blood analyses conducted as part of annual physical examinations. Before 2009, it was the most common test used for diagnosing diabetes and is still relied upon by many doctors and health care facilities.

If you have had an FPG test, you probably haven't forgotten it, especially if you love breakfast. As the name implies, the test measures how much blood sugar is in your system when your stomach is empty. Every-

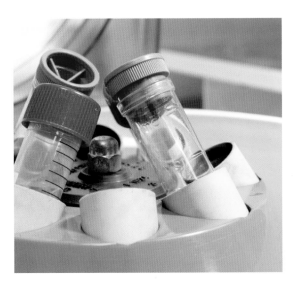

one's glucose spikes after eating a meal, but sugar levels drop within a few hours in people who do not have diabetes. In those with diabetes, blood sugar remains relatively high long after the dishes have been cleared and washed.

If an FPG test is ordered, the patient typically receives instructions not to eat after midnight on the day before the test and then to arrive at a lab bright and early to provide a blood sample. After the blood has been drawn, as the hungry patient bolts for the nearest coffee shop, the lab analyzes the blood. If the test produces a reading lower than 100 mg/dl, diabetes is not present. A reading of 126 mg/dl or higher is a red flag, but since other influences, such as stress and certain illnesses, can raise blood sugar, doctors usually order a retest to confirm the diagnosis.

Inquiring minds may wonder: What if an FPG result is above 100 mg/dl but below 126 mg/dl? If that's the case, the patient has a form of prediabetes called *impaired fasting glucose*. In short, it means the patient doesn't yet have diabetes but may join the club one day. A reading in this middle zone offers a strong clue that insulin resistance has been present for some time.

If any of these tests indicates that a patient's blood sugar is close to normal but the doctor has some reason to suspect diabetes (for instance, if the patient has classic symptoms of the condition), another kind of test may be ordered to clarify matters. An *oral glucose tolerance test (OGTT)* measures how well the body processes sugar that surges into the bloodstream after a meal.

This test is more sensitive than the FBG test, since it does a better job of detecting prediabetes. However, the OGTT takes longer to perform and involves more hassle for the patient. As with the FBG test, it requires that the patient consume nothing but water for eight hours prior to testing. After the patient's blood sugar is measured once, he or she is given a drink containing 75 grams of glucose. Two hours later, a lab technician measures the blood sugar a second time. A result of 139 mg/dl or lower means the patient does not have diabetes. A blood sugar level between 140 and 199 mg/dl is called *impaired glucose tolerance,* a second type of prediabetes. If the reading is 200 mg/dl or higher, the patient is told to come back for a repeat test. A second result above 200 mg/dl indicates diabetes is present.

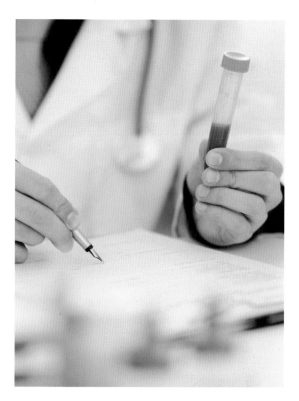

Other tests may be performed to determine the type of diabetes present. High levels of islet-cell antibodies in the blood, low levels of a substance called C-peptide in the blood (which indicates how much insulin the body is making), and high levels of ketones in the urine all indicate type 1 diabetes.

A diagnosis can be scary. However, once you have a diagnosis, you can take steps to put yourself in control of the disease.

GETTING MOTIVATED

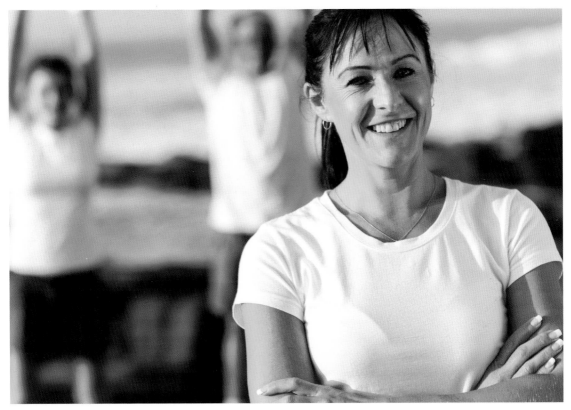

Managing diabetes takes commitment and effort on your part. There may be no better motivation for stabilizing your blood sugar than the fear of living with—or dying from—the devastating long-term complications that are likely to occur if you don't. In this chapter, we give you a glimpse at those potential complications—not only to educate you but also to give you real incentive to walk the path of control. And if the prospect of a bleak future isn't enough to light your diabetes-fighting fire, we also reveal some of the immediate, tangible improvements that can come from reining in your blood sugar.

Think of Your Future

Perhaps you know or have heard of someone who wound up going blind, losing a foot, or needing kidney dialysis because of diabetes. Unfortunately, that's only the tip of the iceberg when it comes to the long-term effects of poorly controlled diabetes. Diabetes can produce a number of serious consequences if you don't take good care of yourself and manage your condition properly.

If the thought of your body decaying and falling apart strikes serious fear into you, *good!* Fear can be a powerful motivator. It's what keeps us from doing stupid things like playing with fire and picking fights with people twice our size. And maybe, just maybe, it will inspire you to control your blood sugar. Some of the proven long-term benefits of quality blood sugar management include:

- improved heart health
- better blood flow
- healthy kidneys
- proper nerve function
- less nerve pain
- fit feet
- clear vision
- mental soundness
- healthy teeth and gums
- flexible joints
- a positive outlook

Improved Heart Health

Despite the long list of health problems diabetes can cause, heart disease is what ultimately kills the majority of people with diabetes. People with diabetes are at least twice as likely to develop heart disease and two to four times more likely to die from it than are people without diabetes. Why? To begin with, many people with diabetes are overweight and have elevated blood cholesterol and blood pressure levels, any one of which on its own increases the risk of heart disease. But diabetes itself is considered a major risk factor for heart disease because having excess sugar in the bloodstream threatens the heart. Sugar is a sticky substance that makes cholesterol, fat, and other substances in the blood stick to the interior walls of blood vessels, contributing to the formation of plaque. Plaque makes blood vessels thick and inflexible, a condition known as atherosclerosis, or hardening of the arteries. The thickening of the blood vessel walls narrows the space through which the blood flows, slowing its passage. And sometimes pieces of plaque break off, which may lead to the formation of blood clots that further restrict the flow of blood to vital organs such as the heart.

The good news: Improving blood sugar control dramatically reduces the risk of heart disease. In addition to preventing the formation of much of the plaque that clogs blood vessels, better diabetes management also frequently leads to reductions in blood cholesterol and blood pressure levels.

Plus, the positive lifestyle steps you take to control blood sugar, such as exercising regularly, eating more healthfully, and cutting back on stress, further reduce your risk of heart disease.

Better Blood Flow

In addition to the heart, a number of other vital body parts require large amounts of oxygen and depend on healthy blood vessels to deliver an unobstructed flow of oxygen-rich blood. The most important of these is the brain. When a blood vessel leading to the brain becomes clogged with sticky plaque, the brain cells normally fed by that vessel do not receive enough oxygen and quickly die. This is called a stroke. The risk of stroke is two to four times higher in people with diabetes than in people who do not have it.

The muscles in the legs also depend on a reliable and substantial flow of blood. When blood vessels that feed the legs become clogged, the leg muscles don't get sufficient oxygen, which can lead to pain or cramping during exercising or walking. This condition is called claudication. Blood vessel disease in the legs is *20 times* more common in people with diabetes than in those without it. Claudication occurs in 15 percent of people who have had diabetes for 10 years and 45 percent of those who have had it for 20 years.

The good news: Tightening blood sugar control, along with all the other changes and lifestyle improvements that come with it, will help blood flow more freely to all the vital body parts. For people with diabetes who have already developed circulatory problems,

symptoms often decrease as blood sugar levels improve.

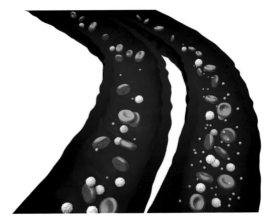

Normal vs. Diabetes blood stream

Healthy Kidneys

Visit any kidney dialysis center and check the charts of the people who sit there for hours a day, several days a week, with tubes in their arms, hooked up to machines that filter waste products, toxins, and other undesirable substances from their blood. Most are diabetic.

Diabetes is the leading cause of kidney failure, accounting for 44 percent of new cases of kidney disease. More than 200,000 Americans with diabetes have received kidney transplants or are receiving dialysis treatment. Approximately 50,000 Americans with diabetes begin treatment for end-stage renal (kidney) disease each year. Minorities, especially African Americans and Hispanics, who have type 2 diabetes are highly susceptible to kidney disease, but everyone with elevated blood sugar levels is at risk. Elevated blood sugar damages the tiny blood vessels, called capillaries, which form and nourish the filters within the kidneys.

The good news: Tightening blood sugar control dramatically reduces the risk of kidney disease. In fact, major studies examining the effect of blood sugar levels on kidney disease found that every 30 mg/dl drop in average blood sugar leads to a 30 percent reduction in the risk of kidney disease.

Proper Nerve Function

The nervous system is like the body's electrical wiring, relaying signals that control voluntary and involuntary functions throughout the body. A portion of that interior wiring, called the autonomic nervous system, controls the body's involuntary activities. Those activities include all of the basic, "behind the scenes" functions—such as the beating of the heart, the digestion of food, the regulation of body temperature, the maintenance of balance, and the physical response to sexual stimulation—that occur without conscious thought or direction on our part.

Nerves are like any other living tissue in the body: They use sugar for energy, and they require an unobstructed blood supply to provide them with oxygen and other nutrients. Excess sugar in the blood appears to cause two main problems for the nervous system. First, it interferes with the blood supply to the nerves—just as it interferes with the flow of blood to other parts of the body—by contributing to plaque buildup in the blood vessel walls. Second, high blood sugar seems to alter energy metabolism (the process of using sugar to fuel cell functions) in such a way that the nerves swell and the coating on the outside of the nerve fibers fails to do its job

of insulating and protecting the nerves. When the nerves that regulate basic body functions are damaged in this way by high blood sugar levels, the condition is referred to as autonomic neuropathy.

Population-based studies have shown that 60 to 70 percent of people with diabetes have some form of mild to severe nerve damage. For example, nearly 50 percent of all men with diabetes develop impotency within a decade of diagnosis, due mainly to malfunction of the nerves that produce an erection. Men who suffer from diabetes also tend to develop problems with erectile dysfunction as much as 10 to 15 years earlier than men who don't have diabetes. Women with diabetes are more likely than women without it to suffer from vaginal dryness, again as a result of damage to nerves that control sexual response. One study found that 18 percent of women with type 1 diabetes and 42 percent of those with type 2 experienced sexual dysfunction.

Nerve damage can also lead to delayed digestion, a condition known as gastroparesis that affects an estimated 25 to 55 percent of people with diabetes (30 percent of those with type 2), especially those who spent many years with uncontrolled blood sugar. Gastroparesis can cause painful bloating and, because it delays the peaking of blood sugar that normally occurs after a meal, can make diabetes even harder to control.

Postural hypotension, yet another condition caused by damage to nerves, is twice as common in people with diabetes. It is a type of low blood pressure that occurs during abrupt changes in position, such as standing up quickly from a seated or prone position, and can lead to dizziness and fainting.

The good news: Blood sugar control is an effective means of preventing all forms of autonomic neuropathy. And while autonomic neuropathy is not always reversible once it has developed, the condition may regress slightly or at least won't progress as quickly once blood sugar levels are returned to normal.

Less Nerve Pain

As previously mentioned, 60 to 70 percent of all people with diabetes develop some form of nerve damage in their lifetime. Of those, most develop a form called peripheral neuropathy— malfunction of the nerves serving the limbs, especially the lower legs and feet. In its early stages, peripheral neuropathy expresses itself as tingling or numbness. But as it progresses and nerves become inflamed, it can cause constant and sometimes severe pain. While there are several conventional and alternative medical treatments for painful neuropathy, many sufferers find little or no relief.

The good news: Tight blood sugar control can help to minimize the pain and slow the progression of peripheral neuropathy. Even better, if it is initiated early enough in the course of diabetes, tight control may actually prevent peripheral neuropathy from developing in the first place.

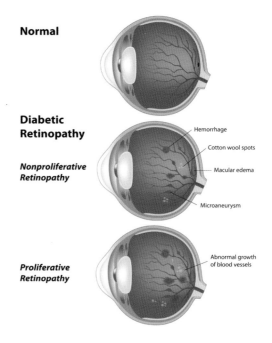

Normal

Diabetic Retinopathy

Nonproliferative Retinopathy

Hemorrhage

Cotton wool spots

Macular edema

Microaneurysm

Proliferative Retinopathy

Abnormal growth of blood vessels

Clear Vision

In the back of the eye is a sensitive layer of tissue called the retina that acts much like the film in a camera. The retina receives and records light from the outside world. Those images in light are then converted into electrical signals that are transmitted to the brain to produce vision. A network of capillaries provides the living cells of the retina with oxygen and nutrients. Elevated blood sugar levels, however, weaken these tiny blood vessels. As a result, they may swell, leak, or grow in unhealthy ways, blocking light from ever reaching the retina. This condition is called diabetic retinopathy.

Diabetes is the leading cause of new cases of blindness among adults ages 20 to 74. Diabetic retinopathy accounts for 12,000 to 20,000 new cases of blindness each year. In fact, roughly one of every five people with type 2 diabetes already has retinopathy when they are diagnosed with diabetes. Glaucoma, cataracts, and diseases of the cornea (the transparent outer covering of the eyeball) are also more common in people with diabetes and contribute to the high rate of blindness among this population.

The good news: Tight blood sugar control reduces the risk of retinopathy. Every 30 mg/dl reduction in average blood sugar lowers the risk of retinopathy by approximately 30 percent. For those with existing retinopathy, tightening blood sugar control slows the progression significantly.

Mental Soundness

With aging comes increased risk for a number of health problems. Few instill as much fear as Alzheimer's disease, a progressive and ultimately fatal disease that destroys brain cells, causing increasingly severe problems with memory, thinking, and behavior along the way. Today, it affects more than five million Americans and is the sixth-leading cause of death in the United States. Currently, there is no cure for Alzheimer's. Damaged blood vessels in the brain are believed to play a role in the development of Alzheimer's. And recent research suggests that people with diabetes are more than twice as likely to develop Alzheimer's compared to those with normal glucose tolerance.

The good news: If you have type 2 diabetes, tight blood sugar control can reduce your risk of Alzheimer's disease to that of the general nondiabetic population.

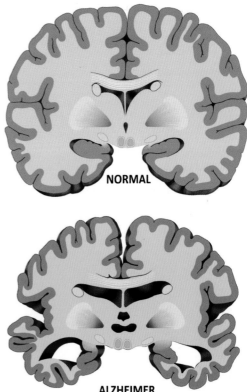

NORMAL

ALZHEIMER

Healthy Teeth and Gums

Adults with diabetes have two times the risk of developing gum disease (periodontitis) as do their peers without diabetes. Almost one-third of people with diabetes have severe gum disease. Specifically, those with type 2 diabetes have greater plaque buildup and more bacteria below the gumline; as a result, their gums bleed more easily, and they commonly experience loosening and loss of teeth. Once a gum infection starts, it can take a long time to eradicate it when blood sugar is out of whack. Conversely, research has shown that having periodontal disease may make it more difficult for people who have diabetes to control their blood sugar levels.

The good news: Good blood sugar control can help prevent dental problems. The lower the average blood sugar level, the lower the risk of gum disease and tooth loss.

Flexible Joints

Joint mobility problems, including conditions such as frozen shoulder, trigger finger, and clawing of the hand, affect approximately 20 percent of people with diabetes, and high blood sugar is the root cause. Excess sugar in the blood sticks to collagen, a protein found in bone, cartilage, and tendons. When collagen becomes sugar-coated, it thickens and stiffens, preventing joints from moving smoothly through their full range of motion and often causing joint pain.

The good news: Keeping your blood sugar levels near normal reduces your risk of developing joint mobility problems. And if you already have limited range of motion in your shoulders, hands, fingers, or other joints, lowering your blood sugar levels may help improve your range of motion and limit the pain associated with stiff joints.

A Positive Outlook

Blood sugar levels have a direct effect on our mental well-being. It's common for people with diabetes to feel down when their blood sugar levels are up. Depression is three to four times more common in adults with diabetes than in the general population. The mechanism of this increased risk is not entirely known. Since depression is often biochemical in nature, elevated sugar levels in the brain may play a direct role. It could also be related, at least

in part, to the extra stress associated with living with a chronic illness. Certainly, developing complications from diabetes can instill a feeling of helplessness, a definite contributing factor in the onset of depression.

The good news: Improving your blood sugar levels can make you a happier person. Researchers at Harvard Medical School and the Joslin Diabetes Center studied the effects of blood sugar control on mood and disposition. They found that people with lower blood sugar levels reported a higher overall quality of life. Significantly better ratings were given in the areas of physical, emotional, and general health and vitality.

Focus on the Immediate Gains

The long-term effects of diabetes and the long-term benefits of improved blood sugar control may indeed help inspire you to start taking your disease more seriously. But what really tends to motivate most people is immediate gratification. These are some of the concrete ways in which you will be rewarded right away for getting your blood sugar levels under control:

- increased energy
- more restful sleep
- improved physical performance
- decreased appetite
- heightened brain power
- more stable moods and emotions
- fewer sick days
- softer skin and healthier gums
- greater personal safety

To provide yourself with powerful reasons to begin managing your diabetes today, try focusing on the many impressive benefits that start coming your way as soon as you start corralling your runaway blood sugar levels.

Increased Energy

Raise your hand if you like being tired all the time. Okay, raise your hand if you're too tired to raise your hand. Elevated blood sugar reduces your overall energy level. Remember, high blood sugar is a sign that not enough sugar is getting into your body's cells, where it is used for energy. The fuel is there; it's just stuck in the bloodstream, kind of like a fleet of gasoline trucks that drive around aimlessly instead of unloading at your local gas station. This shortage of fuel inside the body's cells causes sleepiness and sluggishness. Even if the blood sugar is only elevated temporarily, the lack of energy will be noticeable during that time. As soon as the blood sugar returns to normal, the energy level usually improves. So forget the gimmicky "energy drinks." If you want more energy, control your diabetes!

More Restful Sleep

We all know how important a good night's sleep is to feeling well and being productive the following day. Unfortunately, diabetes makes you more prone to developing sleep disorders, including sleep apnea, a potentially life-threatening disorder in which the sleeper snores loudly and actually stops breathing multiple times throughout the night. Poor blood sugar control also reduces the *quality* of your sleep. If you've ever woken up from a really long night's sleep feeling as though you hardly got any rest at all, it may be because you never reached a deep phase of sleep. Having elevated blood sugar during the night keeps you at a shallow sleep level and prevents you from entering the deep, restful sleep you really need.

If your blood sugar is high enough, you might even wake up several times during the night to run to the bathroom. This is caused by a condition called urine diuresis. When blood sugar reaches more than twice the normal level, some of the sugar spills into the urine, dragging a lot of water along with it. As the bladder fills, it wakes you up. The result may be frequent nighttime urination and even bedwetting. If the thought of a restful, uninterrupted, "dry" night's sleep appeals to you, start getting your blood sugar levels under control now!

Decreased Appetite

It might sound totally backward, but high blood sugar levels tend to make you crave more food—especially carbohydrate-rich food. Remember, when it comes to appetite, it's not the amount of sugar in the bloodstream that counts, it's how much of that sugar gets into the body's cells. If not enough is getting into the cells, particularly the cells that regulate appetite, the body is going to feel hungry no matter how much food is eaten. Given that weight control is so important to both diabetes management and to your long-term health, it makes all the sense in the world to control your diabetes as best you can.

Improved Physical Performance

Elevated blood sugar can reduce your strength, flexibility, speed, and stamina. So whether you're an aspiring athlete or just hoping to make it up a flight of stairs, you can immediately boost your physical abilities by gaining control of your blood sugar.

Muscles prefer sugar as fuel when they make quick, intense movements. When the sugar in the bloodstream can't get into the muscle cells, therefore, strength suffers. Extra sugar in the bloodstream also leads to something called glycosylation of connective tissues, in which sugar coats tendons and ligaments, limiting their ability to stretch properly. Muscle stiffness, strains, and pulls are common in people with high blood sugar levels. High blood sugar also gunks up the connections between muscles and nerves, resulting in dulled reflexes and slower reaction times. And extra sugar in the bloodstream limits the ability of red blood cells to pick up oxygen in the lungs and transport it to working muscles, causing rapid fatigue and restricted cardiovascular/aerobic capacity. So if you want to be able to perform well physically—during sports, exercise, or simple everyday activities—control your diabetes!

Heightened Brain Power

Blood sugar levels influence more than your muscles, ligaments, and tendons. They affect your brain, too. High blood sugar limits your ability to focus, remember, perform complex tasks, and be creative. Studies have repeatedly and consistently shown that mental performance suffers during periods of high blood sugar. As blood sugar goes up, so do mental errors and the time it takes to perform basic tasks. Wide variations in blood sugar levels, from early-morning lows to post-meal spikes, have also been shown to hinder intellectual function. If you (or your loved ones) have noticed a decline in your mental abilities, tightening control of your diabetes might be the answer. Likewise, if you want to perform as well as you possibly can, be vigilant about tracking and balancing those blood sugar levels.

More Stable Moods and Emotions

Besides intellectual performance, your brain is also responsible for maintaining your emotional balance. The fact is, your moods change along with your blood sugar level. Achieving normal blood sugar levels and keeping them there can go a long way toward improving your mood and your emotional stability. That's not to say that you will become an instant optimist or the life of the party. But the way you interact with your family, friends, coworkers, and even perfect strangers truly can impact your success and happiness in life. If you want to be on a more even keel, try evening out your blood sugar levels.

Fewer Sick Days

Bacteria and viruses *love* sugar. They gobble it up and use it to grow and multiply. When blood sugar levels are up, the levels of sugar in virtually all of the body's tissues and fluids rise as well. That makes the diabetic body an ideal breeding ground for infection. If you ignore your high blood sugar levels, therefore, you are essentially supplying extra nutrients to the bad guys. Think of it as aiding and abetting the enemy. Everything from common colds and the flu to sinus infections and vaginal yeast infections are more common when blood sugar levels are elevated. And once illnesses and infections set in, they are much more difficult to shake when blood sugar is high. In fact, people with diabetes are much more likely to die from pneumonia or influenza than are people who do not have diabetes. Research has shown that people who have better blood sugar control spend significantly fewer days absent from work, sick in bed, and restricted from their usual activities. So if you don't like—or can't afford—to get sick, take better care of your diabetes!

Your Body Under Stress

Whether the cause of your stress is physical or emotional, your body will have a response. Stress causes an adrenaline rush, which increases the heart rate, dilates the pupils, tenses the muscles, causes sweating, stops digestion, and makes the liver release a jolt of sugar into the bloodstream for quick energy. In some scenarios, this stress response is a helpful one. If you're under physical threat, quick energy is a good thing! However, we can have the same response to everyday mental stress, and that's less helpful. You don't want your blood pressure, heart rate, and blood sugar level to rise every time you're stuck in rush hour traffic.

The Stress Response and Diabetes

For people with diabetes, managing a stress response can be especially important. The stress hormones that cause the liver to secrete extra sugar into the blood in response to fear, anger, tension, or excitement also increase insulin resistance. For people without diabetes, the stress-induced rise in blood sugar is followed by an increase in insulin secretion, so the blood sugar spike is modest and momentary. For people with diabetes, however, stress can cause blood sugar to rise quickly and stay high for quite a while.

Reducing Stress

We all have some degree of stress in our lives. You can't cut out stress completely. However, you want to minimize its impact on your life. Start by figuring out what causes you stress on an everyday basis, whether it's certain people or common situations. Are there ways you can avoid these stressors? If not, how can you reduce their impact on you?

Minimize interpersonal stress. Unfortunately, other people can cause us lots of stress, and it's useless to try to change other people. With some people, you might want to minimize contact. With others, it is useful to try to understand why they act the way they do, and don't take their actions too personally. Even people whose company we enjoy can cause stress. Think carefully about how you want to spend your time and energy, and don't be afraid to say no to other people's requests for your time or energy.

Take a break. Make time for your hobbies. Take a stroll after dinner. Schedule a massage or aromatherapy session. Go to a concert. Take a scenic drive and turn the music on.

Take advantage of endorphins. Spend some time exercising. Hitting baseballs in a batting cage can be a great form of stress relief! Consider taking up the practice of yoga, pilates, tai chi, or some other form of relaxing movement. Virtually every health club, YMCA, and adult education program offers classes that teach such activities. Many hospitals do, as well.

Get your eight hours of sleep. When we're sleep deprived, we're likely to become stressed more easily. Fatigue can be a source of physical and emotional stress in its own right.

Relax your muscles. Tighten and release your muscles one group at a time, from face to toes, spending about ten seconds on each muscle group. This forces your muscles to relax. Simply knowing how your muscles feel when you are relaxed will make it easier for you to detect when you're feeling tense in response to stress.

WHICH CAME FIRST?

Having diabetes can increase a person's risk of becoming depressed, but research published in 2010 suggests the reverse may also be true—that being depressed can increase one's odds of developing type 2 diabetes. The ten-year study looked at more than 65,000 women who were 50 to 75 years old in 1996. Participants who had diabetes at the start of the study turned out to be nearly 30 percent more likely to develop depression; for those who used insulin to control blood sugar, the likelihood of developing depression was over 50 percent.

But in a bit of a twist, study subjects who were depressed actually had a 17 percent greater chance of developing type 2 diabetes over the course of the study—even after researchers made adjustments for diabetes risk factors such as inactivity and overweight, which also tend to be more common in people who are depressed. The researchers suggested that antidepressant medications as well as the body's own stress hormones—which can affect the body's ability to control blood sugar as well as the way it stores fat—may play some role in the increased diabetes risk.

ASSEMBLING YOUR CARE TEAM

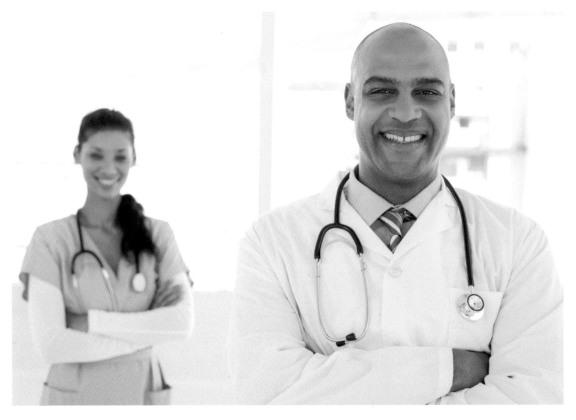

Now that you know a bit more about diabetes in general and why managing it properly is so important, you're probably anxious to start getting your condition under control. But where exactly do you begin, and what will you need to do to succeed?

To get the practical information, personalized advice, treatments, and support you need to begin successfully controlling your diabetes, you need to surround yourself with knowledgeable, experienced, trustworthy experts who can help you: In other words, you need to build your very own diabetes care team.

Recruiting Pros

If you haven't already, find a doctor who not only has skill and experience in diagnosing and treating diabetes, but also one who will support and work with you in becoming the "boss" of your diabetes care. (Yes, that's right: Even though you are assembling a team of diabetes experts, you will ultimately remain responsible for your care. After all, *your* body and *your* future are on the line.) Together you and your doctor need to develop a good working relationship where there is mutual understanding, respect, and trust. You will need to feel comfortable talking honestly and openly with—and asking questions of—your doctor. If you are unable to develop such a relationship, you need to find another doctor.

Look for either an endocrinologist—a physician specially trained to treat people with hormone-related disorders such as diabetes—or an internist or general practitioner who has extensive experience in treating people with diabetes. You can get a list of the doctors in your area by contacting the American Diabetes Association (ADA) at 1-800-DIABETES or visiting their website at www.diabetes.org. If you cannot find a specialist near you, pick a primary care doctor who will work with you and who won't hesitate to refer you to a specialist when one might be needed.

Education is by far the most basic tool of diabetes care. It involves learning how to take care of yourself and your diabetes, and it brings you into the decision-making process for your own health. So after you find a doctor, you'll need to add a certified diabetes educator (CDE) to your team. A certified diabetes educator is a health professional—often a nurse, registered dietitian, exercise physiologist, or pharmacist—who has additional training in helping people with diabetes to manage their disease on a day-to-day basis. Your CDE will provide you with detailed information and one-on-one guidance. As with your doctor, the educator you choose should be someone you feel comfortable talking to and feel you can contact with questions about the practical aspects of diabetes care.

To be certified by the National Certification Board for Diabetes Educators, a health professional must have at least two years and 1,000 hours of experience in diabetes education, be currently employed in a defined role as a diabetes educator for a minimum of four hours each week, and have successfully completed a comprehensive examination covering diabetes. Your physician or health insurance plan may be able to refer you to a certified diabetes educator, or you can contact the American Association of Diabetes Educators at 1-800-338-3633 or visit their website at www.diabeteseducator.org for the names of certified diabetes educators in your area.

In addition, you should stock your diabetes care team with:

- An ophthalmologist (eye doctor), a dentist, and a podiatrist (foot doctor) experienced in treating the specific problems associated with diabetes in their respective fields
- A registered dietitian who has experience in helping people with diabetes to create and adopt a personalized meal plan and make food choices that will improve blood sugar control

- An exercise physiologist who has set up suitable exercise programs for other people with diabetes and worked with them to ensure they are executing the movements and activities safely and effectively
- A therapist, social worker, or other mental health counselor who understands the needs, concerns, and challenges of people living with a chronic disease such as diabetes

Your personal physician may be able to refer you to suitable candidates for these open spots on your diabetes care team. A family member or friend with diabetes may also have suggestions. Otherwise, you can also check the websites of various health and professional organizations; several have search functions that can provide you with the names of qualified members in your area (see the box Wanted: Experts). If you already have an established relationship with an eye doctor, dentist, or podiatrist, be sure to discuss your diabetes diagnosis with them and perhaps even put them in touch with the other members of your team so that they can collaborate on your care.

As you go about assembling your team, remember that these people work for you. You are hiring them to help you learn about diabetes, understand how it specifically affects you, and provide you with the tools to help you successfully manage your disease.

WANTED: EXPERTS

You can visit the websites of the organizations listed below to locate health professionals in your area who can assist you in properly managing your diabetes.

American Academy of Ophthalmology
www.aao.org
American Association of Clinical Endocrinologists (AACE)
www.aace.com
American Dental Association (ADA)
www.ada.org
Academy of Nutrition and Dietetics
www.eatright.org
American Podiatric Medical Association (APMA)
www.apma.org
American Society of Exercise Physiologists (ASEP)
www.asep.org

Keep Your Team Informed

Once you've assembled your diabetes care team, it's important that you keep them on the same page by providing them with up-to-date information on your blood sugar levels, treatment plan, other medical problems, medications, and so forth. A great way to do this is by creating your own medical chart, much the way a doctor or hospital keeps a chart for each patient. This way, you can have all the information about your diabetes and your health in one place, and you can take it with you each time you meet with a member of your diabetes care team.

You'll find a list of the types of information your chart should contain in the box For Your Record. It is particularly crucial that your chart include a complete, accurate, and up-to-date list of all of your medications and the strength and dosage of each. Be sure to include all prescription drugs and any nonprescription medications, vitamins, minerals, supplements, and natural products you take—whether for diabetes or for any other condition/reason. It is important that each member of your care team (and any other medical professional you visit, for that matter) knows what the others have prescribed and what over-the-counter products you take so that together you can avoid dangerous interactions and overdoses. It is also important for *you* to know what you are taking, why you are taking it, and what side effects or warning signs may occur. It is, after all, your body, and you shouldn't put anything in it that you don't understand. Be sure to note in your chart any side effects or unusual symptoms you experience that you suspect may be connected to your medications; then be sure to inquire about them the next time you talk to the prescribing doctor.

It's also very helpful to keep a running list of questions you have about diabetes and/or your treatment plan so that you can query the appropriate team member at your next appointment. Jot down questions or concerns in your chart as they occur to you rather than assuming you'll remember them when you meet with a team member. Often, due to the pressure of limited time or nervousness, you may forget questions that seemed so clear in your mind before you arrived for your appointment.

In addition, take time to prepare for each visit the day prior to your appointment. Be sure to bring your chart as well as your blood glucose meter and any additional logs or records you keep.

FOR YOUR RECORD

Here are the elements to include in the personal medical chart that you maintain:

- A list of your medicines; their strengths; how, when, and why you take them; and who prescribed them

- A list of your medical conditions and dates of diagnosis, any drug or other allergies, and all major medical events and surgeries

- The names, specialties, and contact information—including emergency numbers—for all of the health care professionals you work with

- Any laboratory test results as well as all handouts, booklets, or instructions given to you by members of your diabetes care team

- A running list of questions you have for members of your diabetes care team (with space to record the answers)

Include Family and Friends

Diabetes is sometimes referred to as a family disease, because it tends to affect every family member—and often, close friends—to some extent. It may alter food selection and preparation and timing of shared meals. It may affect leisure time (less TV, more physical activity). It may affect finances. And it's likely to spark an array of emotions—from concern to resentment.

It's also likely to prompt many questions, some you may not care to answer. ("Should you be eating that?" "Why do you have to check your blood sugar so much?" "Did you get diabetes from eating too much sugar?" "Can I catch it from you?") Still, do your best to answer them, and when you can't, ask members of your diabetes care team if they can provide you with the needed information. The more your family and friends know about your disease, the more likely they will be to accept and support your management efforts. The less they know, the more likely they will misunderstand or even unwittingly sabotage your efforts. So show off your knowledge! Teach them as much as you can about diabetes, encourage them to voice their questions and emotions, and involve them in your quest for good control. Share your treatment plan with them, explain why meal planning and blood testing are so vital to your care, tutor them on how to recognize and react to signs of hypoglycemia (which you'll learn about in chapter 9: Avoiding Highs and Lows), and provide concrete suggestions for how they

can support you. You might even consider encouraging them to join you in some of the healthier lifestyle choices you are making. After all, many of the diet and exercise adjustments you'll be making—like becoming more active, cutting down on junk food and other empty calories—can be beneficial for everyone, not just those who have diabetes.

At the same time, keep in mind that this is *your* diabetes, *your* health, *your* life—not theirs. If they aren't interested in joining or even supporting you, let them do what they want—it's not your job (nor is it possible, for that matter) to change the way others live their lives. All you can do is make the right choices for yourself. And if you are concerned about how others will view you for adopting a healthier lifestyle, stop worrying. Deep down, everyone respects and admires those who make the tough choices and take good care of themselves, as long as they don't try to force their beliefs on others.

So the next time your family comes together for a holiday, don't hesitate to get up from the sofa and politely ask, "Anyone care to join me for a walk?" If nobody joins you, that's okay. Maybe next time someone will be inspired by what you're doing and tag along. And when you get together with your friends for a game of bridge or rummy, remember that there is no rule stating that you must consume a handful of snacks for every hand of cards. Have fun, and enjoy the camaraderie and challenge of the game. Just do so without stuffing yourself!

TRACKING YOUR BLOOD SUGAR

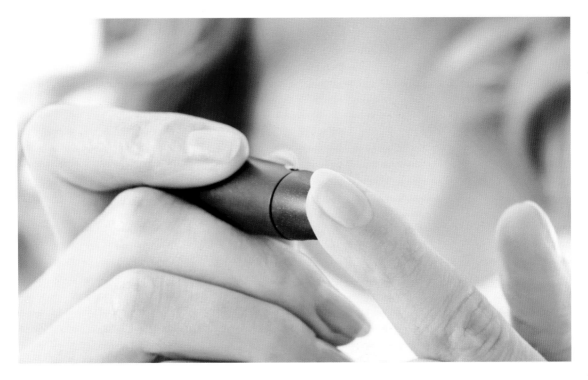

To successfully manage your diabetes and minimize your risk of suffering diabetes complications, you need to do a topnotch job of controlling your blood sugar. But how do you even know what your blood sugar level is at any given point in time? Or how much it varies from day to day and week to week? Or whether the steps you take to get your blood sugar under control are actually working? You use two monitoring methods: individual blood sugar readings and blood tests of a substance called HbA1c.

In this chapter, we explore these two important methods for tracking your blood sugar. We look at what they can tell you about your disease management and how you can use them to improve your blood sugar control. We help you set blood sugar goals that reflect a level of control appropriate for you. And we go through the practical aspects of testing your blood sugar.

Evaluating Your Control

Monitoring your blood sugar when you have diabetes or even prediabetes is very much like paying attention when you drive. You look ahead, behind, and to the sides so you can assess the conditions of the road and avoid other cars. You steal quick glances at the speedometer so you can maintain a safe speed and avoid costly tickets (and accidents). And you heed the various warning lights on the dashboard so you'll know when it's time to take your vehicle in for fuel, maintenance, or repairs.

Ignoring your blood sugar levels, on the other hand, is like driving with a blindfold on. Sooner or later, you're going to crash.

To properly manage your diabetes, you'll have to make many important choices every day. To avoid "driving blind" as you make those choices, you need to be able to "see" where your blood sugar level is and how it's been behaving in response to your "course adjustments." To gain these essential insights, you need to test your blood sugar levels often and have HbA1c tests performed regularly. Of course, you also need to have an idea of where you want to end up—in other words, where your blood sugar levels should be to give yourself the best chance of avoiding devastating diabetes complications. And that means setting goals.

Individual Blood Sugar Readings

Individual blood sugar readings are essential for evaluating your blood sugar control (or lack thereof). These are the readings you get by pricking your finger (or, depending on the equipment you use, an alternate site such as your arm or leg) and placing the resulting drop of blood on a test strip, which you then insert into a portable blood glucose meter. The meter then measures and reports your current blood sugar level.

Regularly gathering, recording, and reviewing your individual blood sugar "numbers" in this way serves several important purposes: **(1)** It provides a measuring stick for assessing your current state of blood sugar control. **(2)** It lets you track your progress from one point in time to another. **(3)** It reveals where improvements need to be made. **(4)** It teaches you the impact of your daily activities and choices. You can see, almost immediately, what works and what doesn't when it comes to keeping your blood sugar in a healthy range. Such prompt feedback not only provides you with a tool for tracking your control, it allows you to take action at once to bring a high or low level back into a healthier range.

Your blood sugar levels naturally vary throughout the day and from day to day, depending on a variety of factors, such as when you ate your last meal, exercised, and took any prescribed diabetes medication. By taking multiple readings each day and then averaging together all of the readings from the last one or two weeks, you can get additional insight into your level of control. Indeed, some glucose meters automatically calculate the average of your recent readings for you.

However, *quality* blood sugar control doesn't just mean having the lowest average. It also

| **Tim:** | 113, 97, 120, 135, 144, 100, 177, 83, 111 | 120 |
| **John:** | 53, 204, 188, 67, 170, 68, 80, 202, 48 | 120 |

requires stability, because blood sugar readings that bounce from high to low aren't healthy, even when they result in an average that doesn't look so bad. Consider, for example, the blood sugar readings of two people, Tim and John.

You can see in the table at the top of the page, both men have the same average blood sugar level. But look at the *variation* in John's readings: His blood sugar is high half the time and low half the time. Tim's blood sugar levels, on the other hand, are more stable and consistent, with no wild upward or downward spikes.

Too much variability in blood sugar levels can affect a person's quality of life. Having an episode of low blood sugar can be dangerous as well as uncomfortable, because it can cause symptoms such as dizziness, weakness, and rapid heartbeat; left untreated, it can quickly lead to blurred vision, confusion, loss of consciousness, and coma. Experiencing such risky lows on a regular basis is like living life on a tightrope. A high level of blood sugar, conversely, saps energy and mental focus, and frequent highs can become a real drag on the body and mind. There is also evidence that excessive variability in blood sugar levels can cause damage to blood vessels, even if the overall average is within the preferred range.

The preferred, or ideal, range for your blood sugar level depends on your current diabetes treatment regimen and how likely it is to cause hypoglycemia, or low blood sugar. That ideal range also varies based on when you take a reading—your ideal range will be different after a night of fasting than it will be an hour or two after a meal, for example. You can use the table on page 40 to determine your ideal fasting, pre-meal, and post-meal ranges. Once you know them, you can assess the quality of your blood sugar control by considering how often your readings fall within the appropriate ranges.

It is not necessary for your blood sugar to be in your ideal range every time you check it. Every person who has been diagnosed with diabetes has moments of weakness when it comes to managing the disease. As a general rule, if at least 75 percent (three out of four) of your readings are in the proper range, you're doing a pretty good job of controlling your blood sugar. If more than 10 percent (one out of ten) of your readings are below your ideal range or if more than 25 percent (one out of four) are above it, you may need some additional self-management education or an adjustment to your medication regime.

Consider Irene, for example. She does not take any medication that can cause hypoglycemia, so her ideal pre-meal range is 70 to 120.

IDEAL BLOOD SUGAR RANGES

	Fasting (Wake-Up) Range	Pre-Meal Range	Post-Meal Range (1–2 hours after eating)
No risk of hypoglycemia*	70–100 mg/dl	70–120 mg/dl	<140 mg/dl
Low risk of hypoglycemia**	70–120 mg/dl	70–140 mg/dl	<160 mg/dl
High risk of hypoglycemia***	70–100 mg/dl	80–160 mg/dl	<180 mg/dl

mg/dl means milligrams per deciliter

* Includes those who are not taking insulin or medications that can cause hypoglycemia (glyburide, glipizide, meglitinides).

** Includes those taking insulin once daily or oral medications that can cause hypoglycemia (glyburide, glipizide, meglitinides).

*** Includes those taking multiple insulin injections daily and those unable to detect hypoglycemia.

The table to the right shows Irene's pre-meal blood sugar readings for five days. Out of 20 readings, none is below her ideal range, which is good; however, 10 are above the upper limit of 120. That means 50 percent of her readings are above her ideal range. So Irene needs to work on tightening her pre-meal blood sugar control.

MON	TUE	WED	THU	FRI
104	174	138	97	86
225	126	125	101	99
166	213	159	110	90
113	98	79	185	143

If your current blood sugar readings are well above your ideal ranges, it's reasonable to set temporary targets that fall between the two. For example, if you are not at risk for hypoglycemia but have blood sugars that are consistently above 200, an initial goal might be to get your readings into the 100 to 180 range. Once you've brought your sugar levels down into that target range, you can then aim for your ideal range(s).

HbA1c Measurements

The second essential tool for gauging your blood sugar control is a test that measures glycohemoglobin A1c, often referred to as HbA1c or simply A1c. The result of this simple blood test, arranged through your doctor's office, reflects your average blood sugar level over the previous two to three months, giving you insight into your blood sugar control over a longer term.

Inside your red blood cells is a protein called hemoglobin that carries oxygen from your lungs to your body's tissues. Sugar in the blood has a tendency to glycate, or stick to, this protein, forming glycohemoglobin. Once the glucose attaches to the hemoglobin, it stays there as long as the red blood cell lives, typically two to three months. Your red blood cells don't all die at once; old ones are constantly dying, and new ones are constantly being created. So at any one time, your red blood cells are a mix of the very old, the middle aged, and the quite young.

In someone without diabetes, roughly 4 to 6 percent of their hemoglobin is coated with sugar. In the person with diabetes, whose blood sugar levels are higher, more sugar attaches to the hemoglobin molecules; usually anywhere from 6 to more than 20 percent of the hemoglobin is sugar-coated. The A1c test measures this percentage. (A1c, by the way, refers to a type of glucose-coated hemoglobin that is especially suited for gauging long-term blood sugar levels.) And because some of the hemoglobin molecules in the blood are older and some newer, the A1c result provides a good estimate of how high the blood sugar has been over the past two to three months.

That's why you should ask your doctor to order an A1c test for you every three months until your sugar levels and A1c are stable and within your target ranges. Once you've reached those goals, it's usually sufficient to have the A1c test every six months, unless your doctor orders more frequent testing.

It's true that several companies sell at-home A1c test kits, but you're probably better off having a professional draw your blood and send it to a laboratory for testing. (Many doctors' offices and virtually all hospitals can do this for you.) Although the at-home kits are reasonably accurate, they require multiple steps. If any of the steps are not performed exactly right, the test will be useless and you'll have wasted your money on the cost of the kit. You may just want to let the professionals handle this test.

When you use the results from the A1c and the individual blood sugar tests you perform yourself, you get a fuller and more accurate picture of your level of control. Using the individual results alone would be like trying to judge a baseball batter's ability by looking at a day or two of single at-bats. Just as a great hitter will make an out or have a bad day sometimes, a person with good control will have the occasional high or low. So to truly gauge the player's batting skill, you need to also see his season average. And to evaluate your level of sugar control, you need to know your A1c.

To translate your A1c result into an average blood sugar level, you can use the following formula:

$$(A1c \times 28.7) - 46.7 = \text{average blood sugar}$$

Or, if math isn't your thing, just use the table at the top of the next page.

A1C	AVERAGE BLOOD SUGAR
5%	97
6%	126
7%	154
8%	183
9%	212
10%	240
11%	269
12%	298
13%	326
14%	355

There's another reason testing A1c is so important. Research has shown it is closely linked to the risk of developing diabetic complications. Essentially, the higher the A1c, the greater the risk of developing eye, kidney, nerve, and heart problems. That is why you should try to keep your A1c as near to normal as possible. In most cases, that equates to an A1c of 6 to 7 percent.

A looser A1c of 7 to 8 percent, however, may be a more appropriate target for anyone in whom an episode of hypoglycemia would be especially dangerous, including:

- Anyone who is susceptible to low blood sugar but suffers from hypoglycemia unawareness, a condition in which the individual is unable to detect the warning symptoms of a dropping blood sugar level until it is too late for them to help themselves; it can develop in people who have had diabetes for many years.

- Anyone who has significant heart disease, because the rapid heartbeat and overall physical stress placed on the body during an episode of hypoglycemia can be particularly dangerous for a person who has an already weakened heart.

- Anyone who works in an extremely high-risk profession (taxi driver, trucker, construction worker, etc.), where experiencing dizziness, blurred vision, confusion, or loss of consciousness due to hypoglycemia could be devastating.

- A very young child who cannot communicate symptoms of hypoglycemia.

On the other hand, a tighter A1c target of 5 to 6 percent may be appropriate for women who are pregnant or preparing to become pregnant, individuals planning for surgery, and anyone looking to slow or reverse existing diabetes complications.

Keep in mind that achieving these A1c targets may take time, especially if your current A1c is very high. Since the test is usually done every three months, it is reasonable to aim for an A1c that's one or two percentage points lower at each test.

Your Specific Target Ranges

When you put it all together, your ideal aim is to have the lowest possible individual blood sugar and A1c levels without experiencing frequent or severe hypoglycemia. Occasional, mild episodes of low blood sugar are acceptable and not dangerous for most people with diabetes. But if low blood sugars become too frequent (occurring more than two or three times a week) or severe (causing seizures or loss of consciousness), you'll need to ease up on your targets. So before proceeding, you need to set your own specific targets, using the information just discussed. Be sure to discuss those targets with your doctor and other members of your diabetes care team. Set targets for the following:

- Blood sugar, fasting range (upon waking)
- Blood sugar, pre-meal range (right before eating)
- Blood sugar, post-meal range (1–2 hours after eating)
- Your A1c target

Testing Your Own Blood Sugar

Okay, you've set your sights on controlling your blood sugar levels. You've even specified exactly where you want your levels to be. Now it's time to prepare for individual blood sugar testing.

Testing Supplies

To perform the individual blood sugar monitoring that is so essential to good control, you need three main supplies: **(1)** a blood glucose meter, **(2)** the testing strips for that meter, and **(3)** a lancet or lancing device to draw the small amount of blood

you'll need for testing. You will also need instruction in using the supplies you choose. Your doctor, certified diabetes educator, and/or pharmacist can give you a hands-on demonstration to ensure that you are using your equipment properly. Meter manufacturers also typically have hotlines that consumers can access in order to get answers and advice about their specific meters. Take advantage of these resources so that you can confidently and correctly measure your blood sugar levels as often as necessary for good control.

When it comes to choosing a meter, remember that quality diabetes management requires accurate and frequent blood sugar testing. Selecting a meter with the desirable qualities listed below should help make *frequent* testing less of a hassle.

- Fast (some meters take just seconds to produce a reading)
- Simple to use (fewer steps mean a quicker process and less chance for user error)
- Provides downloadable results (making it quick and easy to share your results with your diabetes care team)
- Requires very little blood (1 microliter or less is ideal)
- Easy to read (especially if you are visually impaired, choose a meter with a very large display or one that "talks")

The accuracy of just about every blood sugar meter on the market is pretty good. The values these meters produce typically fall within 15 percent of the reading a laboratory would produce on a blood sample taken at the same time. That's true, however, only if you use the correct testing technique. See the Common Testing Problems table for some of the more common monitoring miscues.

With the advent of alternate-site testing—using meters that can test blood taken from places other than the sensitive fingertips, such as the forearm—blood sugar testing that's virtually pain free has become a reality. But be aware that alternate-site testing can be difficult with meters that require 1 microliter of blood or more. Also, a reading taken from the arm or leg may lag several minutes behind a reading taken from the fingertip. So if you suspect that your blood sugar is dropping quickly (after exercise or if you feel hypoglycemic) or rising quickly (after meals), blood taken from your fingertip will provide a more accurate reading than a sample taken from an alternate site.

To make it more likely that you will perform the frequent blood sugar testing that is so conducive to good control, you may find it helpful to have more than one meter. Having multiple identical meters makes testing more convenient (you can keep one in the kitchen and one in the bedroom, for example, or one at work and one at home) and ensures that if one of your meters isn't functioning or gets misplaced, you will have an equivalent backup available. Some meter companies will even send you an extra meter at no charge in an effort to win your loyalty and keep you purchasing their test strips.

When choosing a device for drawing your blood, you'll also want to opt for features and methods that will encourage—or at least won't discourage—frequent testing. For example:

- Use the thinnest-gauge lancet you can find. (The higher the gauge, the thinner the lancet.) Thin lancets are less painful and cause less scarring than thicker lancets. Change the lancet at least once a day so the tip doesn't become dull.

- Use a lancing pen that allows you to adjust the depth of the stick, and turn it to the lightest possible setting that still produces a sufficient blood sample for your meter.

- For finger-stick testing, prick the side of your fingertip rather than the fleshy pad. To obtain a sufficient blood drop after pricking, "milk" your finger by squeezing it, starting at the base and moving toward the tip.

- Opt for alternate-site testing (using your arm or leg, for example) whenever appropriate. It's almost always less painful than sticking your finger, and readings taken at alternate sites are accurate as long as your blood sugar is not rising or dropping quickly at the time of the blood draw.

Before you go out and buy a meter at a local pharmacy, ask your doctor or diabetes educator if any free samples are available. Most meter manufacturers provide free sample meters for distribution to patients, in the hope that more patients will choose their meters and purchase their test strips for years to come. Most health insurance programs, including Medicare, Medicaid, and private insurance, cover the costs of meters, test strips, and lancets. You might want to consider using a reputable mail-order pharmacy or diabetes

COMMON TESTING PROBLEMS

ISSUE	SPECIFICS	SOLUTION
Insufficient blood	If not enough blood is applied to the test area on the strip, the reading may be artificially low.	Dose the strip adequately, as the meter manufacturer instructs. If you suspect a strip contained too little blood, ignore the result and start over with a new strip.
Improper coding	For most meters, you must enter a code number or chip/strip for each new vial or box of strips. If the meter is not coded for that specific package of strips, the readings may be inaccurate.	Every time you begin a new box or vial of strips, code your meter according to the manufacturer's instructions.
Outdated strips	Using test strips that are outdated may produce inaccurate readings.	Check the expiration date before buying and again before starting a vial or box of strips.
Heat or humidity	Heat and humidity will cause test strips to spoil and produce false readings.	Keep your strips sealed in their packaging and away from extreme temperatures. Do not leave test strips in your vehicle!
Dirt/impurities	Having substances like food or grease on your finger or other test site will impact the readings.	Ensure that your test site is clean when you check your blood sugar.

supply service; such operations will typically coordinate the insurance paperwork and ship your supplies directly to you as needed.

Deciding How Often to Test

When it comes to blood sugar monitoring, nobody wants to do more work than is necessary. At the same time, it's essential that you gather enough data so you can assess the quality of your blood sugar control and do some fine-tuning of your management efforts. It is simply not sufficient to check your blood sugar only once a week or only when you wake up in the morning.

What follows are some testing recommendations that vary based on whether you have been diagnosed with type 2 diabetes or prediabetes as well as on which, if any, diabetes medication you currently use. Find the schedule that applies to your current situation, and review the schedule with your diabetes care team before proceeding.

For those with prediabetes or those at high risk who take no diabetes medications: This testing schedule is for those diagnosed with prediabetes or with a high risk of developing diabetes who do not use any oral or injectable medications or insulin for their condition. Each week, you should test your blood sugar four times: just before breakfast one day, just before lunch another day, just before dinner on a third day, and at bedtime on a fourth day. The following is an example of how you might set up this schedule:

Sunday: No testing required.
Monday: Test before breakfast.
Tuesday: No testing required.
Wednesday: Test before lunch.
Thursday: No testing required.
Friday: Test before dinner.
Saturday: Test at bedtime.

This schedule of testing will help you and your diabetes care team determine if your blood sugar remains in a healthy range throughout the day.

For those with type 2 diabetes who don't take insulin: This testing schedule is for those who have been diagnosed with type 2 diabetes but who do not take any insulin for their condition. This schedule applies whether or not any oral medication or any injectable incretin (exenatide, liraglutide, or pramlintide) is also being used.

Test your blood sugar every other day as follows: just before breakfast and then one to two hours after breakfast on day one, just before lunch and then one to two hours after lunch on day three, just before dinner and then one to two hours after dinner on day five, just before breakfast and one to two hours after breakfast on day seven, and so on. The following is an example of how you might set up this schedule:

Monday: Test before and 1–2 hours after breakfast.
Tuesday: No testing required.
Wednesday: Test before and 1–2 hours after lunch.

Thursday: No testing required.
Friday: Test before and 1–2 hours after dinner.
Saturday: No testing required.
Sunday: Test before and 1–2 hours after breakfast.
Monday: No testing required.

This testing schedule will allow you and your diabetes care team to see if your blood sugar remains normal before and after each of your meals. The wake-up and other pre-meal readings indicate whether your body is able to make enough of its own *basal insulin* (the baseline amount of insulin needed to offset the sugar that's naturally released by the liver between meals to maintain basic bodily functions). The after-meal readings indicate whether your pancreas can make enough *bolus insulin* (the additional burst of insulin needed at mealtimes to offset the carbohydrates from a meal).

For those with type 2 diabetes who take long-acting but not rapid-acting insulin: This testing schedule is for those who have been diagnosed with type 2 diabetes who are currently taking long-acting insulin (glargine, detemir, or NPH) but no rapid-acting (lispro, aspart, or glulisine) or premixed (50/50, 70/30, or 75/25) insulin. This schedule applies whether or not any oral medication or injectable incretin (exenatide, liraglutide, or pramlintide) is also being used.

Test your blood sugar at least twice a day, six days a week, as follows: On the first day, test just before and one to two hours after breakfast; on the second day, test just before and one to two hours after lunch; on the third day, test just before and one to two hours after dinner, and also at bedtime if it follows dinner by more than three hours; and on days four through six, repeat the schedule from days one through three. Take a break from testing on the last day of each week. The following is an example of how you might set up this schedule:

Monday: Test before and 1–2 hours after breakfast.
Tuesday: Test before and 1–2 hours after lunch.
Wednesday: Test before and 1–2 after dinner and at bedtime (if it's more than 3 hours after dinner).
Thursday: Test before and 1–2 hours after breakfast.
Friday: Test before and 1–2 hours after lunch.
Saturday: Test before and 1–2 hours after dinner and at bedtime (if it's more than 3 hours after dinner).
Sunday: No testing required.

This testing schedule will allow you and your diabetes care team to see if your blood sugar remains normal before and after each of your meals.

For those with type 2 diabetes who take premixed insulin twice a day: This testing schedule is for those diagnosed with type 2 diabetes who currently inject premixed insulin (50/50, 70/30, or 75/25) twice each day rather than injecting long-acting (glargine, detemir, or NPH) and/or rapid-acting (lispro, aspart, or glulisine) insulin separately. This schedule applies whether or not any oral medication or injectable incretin (exenatide, liraglutide, or pramlintide) is also being used.

Each day of the week, test your blood sugar upon waking (before breakfast), at midday (before lunch), late in the afternoon (before dinner), and at bedtime. Also, as part of your weekly testing regimen, test your blood sugar one to two hours after breakfast on one day, one to two hours after lunch on another day, and one to two hours after dinner on a third day. The following is an example of how you might set up this schedule:

Sunday: Test before breakfast, before lunch, before dinner, and at bedtime.
Monday: Test before breakfast, 1–2 hours after breakfast, before lunch, before dinner, and at bedtime.
Tuesday: Test before breakfast, before lunch, before dinner, and at bedtime.
Wednesday: Test before breakfast, before lunch, 1–2 hours after lunch, before dinner, and at bedtime.
Thursday: Test before breakfast, before lunch, before dinner, and at bedtime.
Friday: Test before breakfast, before lunch, before dinner, 1–2 hours after dinner, and at bedtime.
Saturday: Test before breakfast, before lunch, before dinner, and at bedtime.

The pre-meal checks are necessary because they allow you and your diabetes care team to evaluate the effectiveness of your insulin doses. The post-meal checks help to determine the optimal timing of your two daily injections.

For those with type 2 diabetes who take insulin at each meal: This testing schedule is for those diagnosed with type 2 diabetes who currently inject rapid-acting insulin (lispro, aspart, or glulisine) at each meal and use long-acting insulin (glargine, detemir, or NPH) to cover their basal insulin needs. (No premixed insulin is used.) This schedule applies whether or not any oral medication or injectable incretin (exenatide, liraglutide, or pramlintide) is also being used.

Each day of the week, test your blood sugar just before every meal; just before your afternoon snack; just before your evening snack or, if you don't eat an evening snack, just before going to bed; prior to exercise; and before driving. Also, one day a week, test your blood sugar one to two hours after breakfast; on another day of the week, test one to two hours after lunch; and on a third day, test one to two hours after dinner. The following is a sample schedule:

Sunday: Test upon waking; before lunch; before your afternoon snack; before dinner; before your evening snack or at bedtime; and before exercising or driving.
Monday: Test upon waking; 1–2 hours after breakfast; before lunch; before your afternoon snack; before dinner; before your evening snack or at bedtime; and before exercising or driving.
Tuesday: Test upon waking; before lunch; before your afternoon snack; before dinner; before your evening snack or at bedtime; and before exercising or driving.

Wednesday: Test upon waking; before lunch; 1–2 hours after lunch; before your afternoon snack; before dinner; before your evening snack or at bedtime; and before exercising or driving.

Thursday: Test upon waking; before lunch; before your afternoon snack; before dinner; before your evening snack or at bedtime; and before exercising or driving.

Friday: Test upon waking; before lunch; before your afternoon snack; before dinner; 1–2 hours after dinner; before your evening snack or at bedtime; and before exercising or driving.

Saturday: Test upon waking; before lunch; before your afternoon snack; before dinner; before your evening snack or at bedtime; and before exercising or driving.

The pre-meal tests are necessary because they allow you and your diabetes care team to evaluate the effectiveness of your insulin doses. The pre-driving and pre-exercise tests

IF YOU HAVE TYPE 1

Blood sugar testing is absolutely essential if you have been diagnosed with type 1 diabetes. For you, it's truly a matter of life and death. Your testing schedule may be similar to the one described in the text for people with type 2 diabetes who take insulin at each meal, but you must work with your diabetes care team to determine the timing and frequency of daily testing that is most appropriate for you, based on a variety of factors, including your current level of control.

are for safety purposes. The post-meal tests help you and your team determine the optimal timing of your insulin doses.

Recording and Analyzing Your Results

To make your testing worthwhile, you need to review and learn from your results. By keeping organized and accurate records of your blood sugar tests and analyzing them on a regular basis, you can gain tremendous insight into your diabetes management program.

At its most basic, your record keeping system should include the date and time of every blood sugar test and the results you obtained from each one. As long as your blood sugar readings are consistently within your target ranges, it is not usually necessary to keep track of anything else. But if some of the readings are above or below target, it becomes necessary to figure out why. Was a high or low reading caused by the consumption of too much or too little food? The wrong type, dose, or timing of medication? An unusual amount of physical activity? Stress? Illness? Every time you use your records to make a sensible adjustment to your treatment regimen (whether in the type, amount, or timing of food, physical activity, or medication), your blood sugar control will get a little bit better.

If you need to figure out why your blood sugar levels are straying outside their target ranges, you will need to record other information in addition to your test results. The same is true if your treatment regimen calls for injecting insulin at mealtimes, an approach that requires you to account for meals and physical activity in determining the correct dose of insulin. In either situation, you will need to record the major factors that influence blood sugar levels, including:

- The type, dose, and timing of any diabetes medication (oral medication, noninsulin injection, and/or insulin)

- The grams of carbohydrate consumed in each meal and snack

- The type and length of exercise and other physical activities performed, such as housework, yard work, shopping, and extended walking

- Stresses that tend to affect blood sugar levels, such as physical illness, menstrual cycles, emotional events, and hypoglycemic episodes

Your log sheets need not be fancy. A ruled notebook with columns and headers penciled in by hand will work just fine.

Learning how to interpret your self-monitoring records is also essential. Otherwise, your records are nothing more than pieces of paper covered with numbers. To get the most from your record keeping, it helps to organize the information so it will be easy to analyze. One way is to line up several days' data in columns so that you can detect blood sugar patterns that occur at particular times of day. If you notice that your blood sugar levels are

consistently high or low at a certain point each day, it's easy to make the right kind of adjustment to bring it back in line.

To see how this works, consider the table showing two weeks of blood sugar test results for Ellie. Ellie has type 2 diabetes and is currently taking no insulin or other medication for her diabetes. Ellie's target blood sugar ranges are:

Fasting (before breakfast): 70–100
Before other meals: 70–120
After meals: <140

Notice how Ellie's pre-meal blood sugars are consistently near normal, but her after-meal readings are generally above her target range. It looks as though Ellie needs to work on managing her post-meal blood sugar, possibly through reduced carb intake at meals, some physical activity after meals, or the addition of a mealtime medication.

Now consider the results shown on the table for Debby. Debby is taking long-acting insulin once a day and oral diabetes medication at each meal. Her target blood sugar ranges are:

Fasting (before breakfast): 70–120
Before other meals: 70–140
After meals: <160

Debby's pre- and post-meal blood sugars are all pretty close to her targets, except for her level first thing in the morning. Debby's dose of long-acting insulin likely needs to be increased, or she needs to reduce her late-night snacking.

When you first begin testing, recording, and analyzing your own blood sugar levels, you should review your readings every couple of weeks. If they are fairly stable and within their target ranges, then monthly record reviews should be enough. But if you detect a pattern of readings that are out of range (above or below), bring them to the attention of your diabetes care team. Working with your team, you should be able to develop an effective solution for any control problem. And as your experience grows, there will likely come a time when you will be able to determine for yourself what minor adjustments to make in your treatment regimen to bring any errant levels back where they belong. (Even then, you'll need regular check-ins with your diabetes care team.)

ELLIE

	Before breakfast	After breakfast	Before lunch	After lunch	Before dinner	After dinner
Mon 3/3	95	166				
Wed 3/5			87	144		
Fri 3/7					77	158
Sun 3/9	99	190				
Tue 3/11			80	133		
Thu 3/13					100	202
Sat 3/15	81	175				

DEBBY

	Before breakfast	After breakfast	Before lunch	After lunch	Before dinner	After dinner	Bedtime
Mon 3/3	188	131					
Tue 3/4			102	122			
Wed 3/5					87	128	104
Thu 3/6	211	135					
Fri 3/7			110	114			
Sat 3/8					85	99	98

Continuous Glucose Monitoring

Another tool in diabetes management technology is continuous glucose monitoring (CGM). Several systems are now available (by prescription) that provide blood sugar readings once every one to five minutes and emit warnings when the sugar level is heading for a high or low. These systems use a sensor, a thin metallic filament inserted just below the skin, to detect sugar in the fluid between fat cells. They come with a spring-loaded device that makes inserting the sensor quick and relatively painless. The information from the sensor is transmitted via radio signals to a receiver that looks like a cell phone. The receiver displays charts, graphs, and an estimate of the current blood sugar level. The transmitter and receiver are reusable, although the sensor filament must be replaced every few days or so, depending on the specific system and the body's ability to tolerate the filament.

CGM devices are generally accurate to within about 15 percent of most finger-stick readings. They generate line graphs that depict sugar levels over the past several hours, allowing the user to detect trends and predict where blood sugar is headed. They use either vibration or a beeping noise to alert the wearer to impending high and low blood sugar levels. And computer or internet-based programs allow for detailed analysis of blood sugar levels over longer intervals of time.

Comparing finger-stick blood sugar testing to CGM is like comparing a photograph to a movie. CGM shows change and movement. It illustrates how virtually everything in daily life influences blood sugar levels. Used just once or twice, CGM can offer insight into the effectiveness of an individual's current diabetes management program. Worn on an ongoing basis, CGM makes it easier to keep blood sugars in range on a consistent basis with less risk of experiencing dangerous highs or lows.

Of course, CGM does have its drawbacks. It can be costly, and many health insurance plans resist covering it for people with type 2 diabetes. A CGM system requires some maintenance and technical know-how, and it's not always the most accurate testing method. It also still requires the user to enter the results from periodic finger-stick readings for calibration purposes, and improperly calibrating the device can lead to erroneous readings. But if CGM sounds interesting to you, don't hesitate to talk to your diabetes care team to gather more information about it.

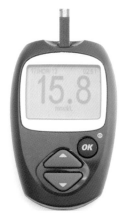

FIGHTING DIABETES WITH FOOD

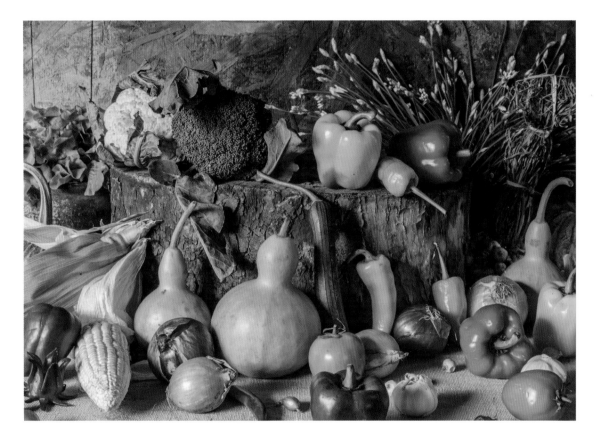

Many people with diabetes assume, especially when first diagnosed, that having diabetes means cutting all the tasty, satisfying foods from their diet. Nothing could be further from the truth. There is no special "diabetic diet" anymore. Rather than a restrictive diet, which can lead to binging on "forbidden" foods, what you need is knowledge and information. You need to understand how food affects your body and then use that information, along with glucose monitoring, to choose a variety of foods—including the ones you enjoy most.

DON'T LABEL FOODS AS GOOD OR BAD

No single food, in and of itself, is good or bad. A chocolate bar, a piece of prime rib, a slice of bread—not one of those is bad, nor does eating one of them mean you've failed somewhere. Even though you have diabetes, each food can fit into your healthy eating plan, as long as you adjust for it. If enjoying it once in a while, in a reasonable portion, keeps you satisfied and out of the common trap of denying yourself foods and then binging on them, then it helps you out in the end.

Control Carbohydrates

Carbohydrates include simple sugars as well as complex carbs. Simple sugars include sucrose (table sugar), fructose (fruit sugar), lactose (milk sugar), and corn syrup. Foods rich in simple carbs include fruit, fruit juice, regular soda, candy, chocolate, cookies, cakes, pastries, milk, ice cream, yogurt, sports drinks, honey, syrup, and jelly.

Complex carbs are better known as starches. Most starches are composed of many sugar molecules linked together. Food rich in starches, or complex carbs, include potatoes, rice, pasta, cereal, oatmeal, bread, pizza, tortillas, bagels, beans, corn, pretzels, chips, and popcorn.

Your body converts the carbs you eat into glucose. To get the sugar out of your bloodstream and into your body's cells, your pancreas produces insulin. Consuming large amounts of carbohydrate places a heavy workload on the pancreas. In people who are insulin resistant or who have a pancreas that has a hard time keeping up, there simply may not be enough insulin produced to keep the blood sugar level from going too high.

For many years, doctors and others advised people with diabetes to avoid simple sugars as much as possible. However, after several conclusive studies, the American Diabetes Association changed its nutritional recommendations. The current understanding is that *from the standpoint of blood sugar control, it doesn't matter if the carbs you eat are simple sugars or complex carbs (starches)*. Both will raise blood sugar by the same amount. A cup of pasta that contains 60 grams of complex carbohydrate will raise your blood sugar just as much as a can of regular soda containing 60 grams of simple sugars.

So how much carbohydrate should you eat? That depends on many factors, including your level of physical activity, your height, and the amount of weight you want to lose. It's something you should discuss with your dietitian.

Once you have an idea of how much total carbohydrate to consume daily, you need to distribute it throughout the day. For example, if you have 160 grams of carbohydrate to "spend" for the day, you could have 30 grams for breakfast, 45 grams for lunch, 20 grams in an afternoon snack, 45 grams for dinner, and 20 grams in an evening snack.

What's a Carb Exchange?

Carb exchanging involves converting food types into grams of carbohydrate. It is based on the traditional, more complex diabetic "Exchange System," which divides foods into categories, such as starches, vegetables, fruits, meats, and so on, with predetermined portion sizes. All food exchanges within a category have roughly equivalent nutritional value and impact on blood sugar levels. For example, one slice of bread counts as one "starch" exchange. It contains about 15 grams carbohydrate, 3 grams protein, and 80 calories. The same can be said of a half cup of cooked pasta, six saltine crackers, a third cup baked beans, or three cups of popcorn. In other words, three cups of popcorn can be "exchanged" for one slice of bread because it contains about the same carb, protein, and calorie count. (You'll find a more detailed exchange list at the back of this book.)

Glycemic Index

Not all carbs are created equal. While virtually all of the digestible carbs you consume will eventually be converted into blood glucose, some make the transition much faster than others. The rate at which different carbs are converted into blood glucose can be compared using something called the Glycemic Index (GI). A food's GI score, therefore, is another factor to take into account when considering the effect a food will have on blood sugar.

The GI ranks foods on a scale from 0 to 100. At the top, with a score of 100, is pure glucose (listed as dextrose on package labels). Other foods are ranked in comparison to the absorption rate of pure glucose. (There's a list of GI scores for many common foods at the back of the book.)

What the score actually represents is the percentage of a food's carbohydrate content that turns into blood glucose within the two hours after the food is eaten.

EXCHANGE GROUP	CARBOHYDRATE	PROTEIN	FAT	CALORIES
1 Starch exchange	15g	3g	Trace	80
1 Fruit exchange	15g	None	None	60
1 Vegetable exchange	5g	2g	None	25
1 Milk exchange	12g	8g	1–8g	90–150
1 Meat exchange	None	7g	3–8g	35–100
1 Fat exchange	None	None	5g	45

- Foods with a high GI score (70 or greater) tend to be digested and converted into glucose the fastest, producing a significant peak in blood sugar 30 to 45 minutes after they are eaten.

- Foods with a moderate GI score (56 to 69) digest a bit slower, resulting in a less pronounced peak in blood sugar approximately one to two hours after they are eaten.

- Foods with a low GI score (55 or less) have a slow, gradual effect on the blood sugar level: The peak is usually quite modest and may take several hours to occur.

Why care about GI scores? Because the effect that different foods have on your blood sugar is what really matters.

Consuming primarily low-GI foods tends to make blood sugar easier to control. A diet of slowly digesting (low-GI) foods eases the workload on the pancreas, prevents post-meal spikes in blood sugar, and provides a satisfying form of slow-burning fuel.

Calories and Weight Loss

The reason people with diabetes must pay such careful attention to calorie intake is that body fat interferes with insulin's action, causing or exacerbating insulin resistance. Each person's daily calorie needs are unique and are based on factors such as height, current weight, ideal weight, metabolism, and physical activity level. As was the case in determining appropriate carbohydrate intake, it is best to seek the guidance of a registered dietitian to help you figure out how many calories you should consume each day.

MEAL	HIGH-GI CHOICES	LOWER-GI CHOICES
Breakfast	Typical cold cereal, bagel, toast, waffle, pancake, corn muffin	High-fiber cereal, oatmeal, yogurt, whole fruit, milk, bran muffin
Lunch	Sandwich made with white or whole-wheat bread, French fries, tortillas, canned pasta	Chili, pumpernickel bread, corn, carrots, raw salad vegetables
Dinner	Rice, rolls, white potato, canned vegetables	Sweet potato, pasta, beans, fresh or steamed vegetables
Snacks	Pretzels, chips, crackers, cake, donut	Popcorn, whole fruit, frozen yogurt

FALLING FOR LESS FAT

If you have diabetes, you need to be concerned about your heart. People with diabetes are three times more likely to develop heart disease. So as you learn to choose healthier foods, it's important to keep your blood cholesterol level and your risk of heart disease in mind. Cutting down the fat in your diet can help improve your blood glucose control, since fat can indirectly elevate your blood glucose levels by blocking the action of insulin. Falling for less fat boils down to choosing more foods that have less total fat and substituting healthier fats for some of the saturated fats you usually eat. Here are some tips:

- Read food labels and opt more often for food with less total fat and less saturated fat.
- Eat a variety of fruits and vegetables, whole-grain products, beans, and nuts. Fruits and vegetables are naturally low in fat and provide loads of nutrients. Whole-grain foods and beans are low in fat but high in nutrients. Nuts, while not especially low in fat, are filled with mostly monounsaturated fats.
- Choose fish more often than poultry; choose poultry more often than red meat.
- Trim visible fat (it's saturated) from meat and fat and skin from poultry before eating.
- Instead of frying, try baking, broiling, roasting, or grilling.
- Use fat-free and low-fat milk products.
- Choose fats and oils that are trans-fat free and have two grams or less of saturated fat per tablespoon.

To lose excess body fat, you must burn more calories than you take in. Increasing your physical activity will help to create a calorie deficit. But exercise alone, with no change in caloric intake, rarely results in significant, sustainable weight loss. Most often, a combination of increased calorie expenditure and a modestly reduced calorie intake leads to the greatest weight loss over the long-term.

Learning to Choose

Unlike dieting, which is all about restrictions, learning to choose healthier foods and eating habits is all about expanding your dietary horizons. Each time you eat becomes an opportunity to choose something lower in salt or fat, something higher in fiber, or food that's richer in vitamins. When you learn to choose, the ball is in *your* court. It is up to *you* how often you make a healthier food choice, how quickly you move toward your goals, and exactly what a healthy, enjoyable diet consists of *for you*.

A diagnosis of diabetes can make the simple act of eating seem overwhelmingly complicated. When you learned you had diabetes, you may have assumed you'd have to go on a special, restrictive diet. But today's dietary approach to managing diabetes focuses on

OPTING FOR LESS SALT

Salt isn't bad—it contains sodium, an essential mineral for the human body. However, too much sodium contributes to high blood pressure, which is especially common in and dangerous for people with type 2 diabetes. Decreasing your salt intake can help reduce your blood pressure, which cuts down on your risk of heart attack, stroke, and kidney problems. Here are some tips on reducing your sodium intake:

- Choose reduced-sodium or no-salt-added products.
- Buy fresh produce; there's no salt added.
- Use fresh poultry, fish, and lean meats more often than canned, smoked, or processed types.
- Try low-sodium versions of soy sauce and teriyaki sauce.
- Use herbs, spices, lemon, lime, vinegar, or salt-free seasoning blends.
- If you like tuna, buy water-packed and rinse the meat to remove some of the salt.
- Take the saltshaker off the table. Always taste your food before adding any salt.
- Choose only small portions of foods that are pickled, cured, in broth, or bathed in soy sauce.
- When dining out, ask that your food be prepared without added salt, monosodium glutamate (MSG), or high-sodium ingredients.
- Limit salty condiments such as ketchup, mustard, pickles, and mayonnaise.

moderation, not deprivation. By trying to completely avoid certain foods, people tend to overconsume them in the end. While people with diabetes need to manage their blood sugar, they can still indulge in a wide variety of tasty foods, including chocolate, peanut butter, popcorn, beef tenderloin, and shrimp. In the pages that follow, we profile an assortment of delicious, nutritious foods you can eat—many of which you may find surprising.

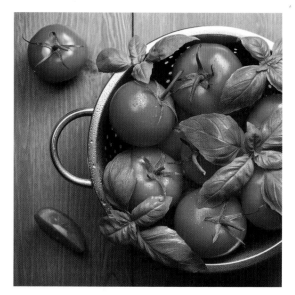

ACORN SQUASH

This acorn-shaped variety of winter squash is full of flavor and nutrients. It's easy to find during fall and winter months and simple to prepare. It's most commonly baked, and its slightly sweet-tasting flesh is high in fiber.

Benefits

Acorn squash is rich in vitamins A (beta carotene) and C and the mineral potassium. Although acorn squash is a starchy vegetable, its high fiber content helps slow the rate that carbohydrates are digested and absorbed, making it a great choice for people with diabetes. Its high potassium level also makes it beneficial for controlling blood pressure.

Selection and Storage

You may find acorn squash year-round, but it's best from early fall to late winter. Look for acorn squash that is deeply colored (dark green with some golden coloring) and free of spots, bruises, and mold. The hard skin serves as a barrier, allowing it to be stored a month or more in a dark, cool place.

Tips

Acorn squash can be baked, steamed, sautéed, or simmered. One of the easiest preparation methods is to cut it in half, scoop out and discard the seeds, and bake it for about an hour. You can serve the baked squash in the skin and fill the center with whatever you like (try rice, barley, pine nuts, and garlic), or you can scoop out the baked flesh and enjoy it mashed or sprinkled with a small amount of Parmesan cheese or other seasonings. Acorn squash is also a tasty addition to savory soups.

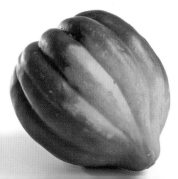

NUTRIENTS PER SERVING:

Acorn squash, ½ cup cooked

Calories: 57
Protein: 1g
Total fat: 0g
Saturated fat: 0g
Cholesterol: 0mg
Carbohydrate: 15g

Dietary fiber: 4.5g
Sodium: 0mg
Potassium: 450mg
Calcium: 45mg
Iron: 9mg
Vitamin A: 439 IU
Vitamin C: 11mg
Folate: 19mcg

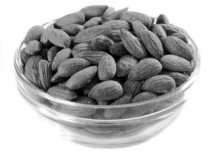

ALMONDS

Although we call them nuts, almonds are actually the seeds of the fruit from an almond tree. We don't eat the outer fruit, but we get a host of nutrients, most notably vitamin E, protein, and healthy, monounsaturated fat, when we munch on tasty almond seeds.

Benefits

Almonds pack a powerful nutrient punch in a small package. Their combination of protein, fiber, and healthy fats makes them a great food that provides lasting energy. They are an excellent source of vitamin E and magnesium and offer calcium and B vitamins, too. Almonds and other nuts are also known to help lower cholesterol levels. Because almonds are calorie-rich, portion control is important.

Selection and Storage

Almonds are available packaged or in bulk, with or without shells. Always check the freshness date on packaged almonds, and if you buy bulk, they should smell fresh. Packaged almonds are available in various forms— whole, blanched (to remove the skin), sliced, slivered, raw, dry or oil roasted, smoked, flavored, and salted or unsalted. Almonds in the shell can keep for a few months in a cool, dry location. Once you shell them or open a package of shelled nuts, they will need to be stored in the refrigerator or freezer.

Tips

Using almonds as a topping or in baking allows you to benefit from their nutrients without overdoing calories. As a snack, stick with a handful, or about 23 almonds (1 ounce). Dry roasted almonds are lower in calories than oil roasted. Enjoy unsalted almonds sprinkled on salads, soups, casseroles, vegetables, stir-fries, cereal, and more.

NUTRIENTS PER SERVING:

Almonds,
1 ounce dry roasted
without salt
Calories: 169
Protein: 6g
Total fat: 15g

Saturated fat: 1g
Cholesterol: 0mg
Carbohydrate: 6g
Dietary fiber: 3g
Sodium: 0mg
Potassium: 200mg

Calcium: 76mg
Iron: 1mg
Folate: 15mcg
Vitamin E: 7mg
Magnesium: 80mg

AVOCADO

Often mistaken for a vegetable, this rich, smooth-textured fruit is most widely recognized when mashed, seasoned, and served as guacamole. Its buttery flavor is a good complement in vegetable, meat, salad, and pasta dishes.

Benefits

Avocados frequently show up on lists of "super foods" for their numerous health benefits. Avocados are rich in monounsaturated fat, a type of fat recommended for a diabetic diet because it can lower LDL (bad) cholesterol, especially when it replaces saturated fat. Still, even the good kind of fat found in avocados is high in calories, so portion control is important. Avocados also contain lutein, a form of carotenoid, an antioxidant that helps maintain healthy eyes and skin. They also contain healthy amounts of fiber, potassium, and vitamins C, K, and B_6.

Selection and Storage

The two most common varieties of avocados are the pebbly textured, dark-colored Haas and the green Fuerte, with its thin, smooth skin. Ripe avocados yield to gentle pressure and should be unblemished and heavy for their size. If you don't plan to use them right away, make sure you choose avocados that are firm. To speed ripening, place avocados in a brown bag on the counter. Once ripened, store in the refrigerator for several days.

Tips

Avocados should be served raw, because they taste bitter when cooked. To use them in a hot dish, add them just before serving. Once avocado flesh is cut and exposed to air, it browns rapidly. Adding the avocado to a dish at the last moment can help minimize this, as can tossing cut avocado with a little lemon or lime juice.

NUTRIENTS PER SERVING:

Avocado, ½ fresh

Calories: 161
Protein: 2g
Total fat: 15g
Saturated fat: 2g
Cholesterol: 0g
Carbohydrate: 9g
Dietary fiber: 6.5g
Sodium: 5mg
Potassium: 485mg
Calcium: 12mg
Iron: 0.5mg
Vitamin A: 147 IU
Vitamin C: 10mg
Folate: 81mcg

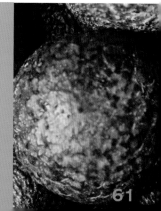

BEEF TENDERLOIN

Surprise! There's no need to ban beef from your diet. Beef tenderloin contains only 8 grams of fat per 3-ounce serving—that's less than a skinless chicken thigh! Considered one of the 29 lean cuts of beef, this tender steak or roast makes for a rich and satisfying meal.

Benefits

Lean beef is highly nutritious, providing quality protein and essential vitamins and minerals. Beef's easily absorbed iron is especially valuable, since a shortage of this mineral is the most common nutritional deficiency and leading cause of anemia in the United States. Half the fat in beef is mono-unsaturated, the same heart-healthy fat in olive oil. And a third of beef's saturated fat is a unique type shown to have a neutral effect on blood cholesterol. Short- and long-term studies indicate lean beef can fit in diets for lowering blood cholesterol.

Selection and Storage

Choose beef with a bright cherry-red or purplish color without any gray or brown blotches. Purchase tightly sealed packages before or on the "sell by" date on the package. Refrigerate or freeze beef as soon as possible after purchase. Use refrigerated beef within four days after purchase. To keep beef tenderloin lean, trim all fat from the exterior. To find other lean beef cuts, look for "loin" or "round" in the name.

Tips

Tender beef cuts, like tenderloin, are best prepared with a dry-heat cooking method, such as roasting, grilling, broiling, or stir-frying. These methods require little or no added fat. When using a marinade, tender cuts need only 15 minutes to 2 hours to add flavor. A seasoning rub is another great way to add flavor to the surface of beef. Cook to an internal temperature of at least 145°F (medium rare) to be safe.

NUTRIENTS PER SERVING:

Beef tenderloin, trimmed of all fat, 3 ounces roasted

Calories: 174
Protein: 23g
Total fat: 8g
Saturated fat: 8g
Cholesterol: 72g

Carbohydrate: 0g
Dietary fiber: 0g
Sodium: 50mg
Potassium: 280mg
Iron: 1.4mg
Zinc: 4.2mg
Phosphorus: 184mg
Vitamin B_6: 0.5mg
Vitamin B_{12}: 1.2mcg

BLUEBERRIES

Blueberries are antioxidant superstars, ranking second among top antioxidant-rich foods. Great for your eyes, memory, and heart, these flavorful berries are a true health bargain.

Benefits

Besides being packed with antioxidants, blueberries are a good source of fiber and provide vitamin C and iron. Recent research suggests that eating blueberries as part of a healthy diet may help reduce several key risk factors for cardiovascular disease and diabetes, such as accumulation of belly fat, high blood cholesterol, and high blood sugar. Antioxidants in blueberries may also protect your eyes and brain cells and help reverse age-related memory loss.

Selection and Storage

Blueberries are at their best when they are in season—from May through October. Choose blueberries that are firm, uniform in size, and indigo blue with a silvery frost. Sort and discard shriveled or moldy berries, but do not wash blueberries until you're ready to use them. Store them in a moisture-proof container in the refrigerator for up to five days. Freeze washed and dried blueberries in a single layer on a cookie sheet, and place in a sealed bag or container once frozen.

Tips

Enjoy blueberries on cereal, in yogurt or salads, with a splash of cream, or simply out of hand. Blueberry jam is a nutritious low-fat spread for toast or crackers. Frozen blueberries make a refreshing snack on a hot day and are a great addition to smoothies. Once frozen, blueberries are best used in baking, as they become mushy once thawed. Blueberries are easy to bake into muffins, pancakes, quick breads, pies, cobblers, and fruit crisps.

NUTRIENTS PER SERVING:

Blueberries, ½ cup raw

Calories: 42
Protein: 1g
Total fat: 0g
Saturated fat: 0g
Cholesterol: 0g
Carbohydrate: 11g
Dietary fiber: 2g
Sodium: 0mg
Potassium: 60mg
Calcium: 4mg
Iron: 0.2mg
Vitamin A: 401 IU
Vitamin C: 7mg
Folate: 4mcg

CASHEWS

The delicately flavored nut is a wise nut choice for people with diabetes. Researchers are studying the potential role of cashew-nut extract in the treatment of the disease.

Benefits

Cashews have long been used in traditional medicine to treat high blood sugar, and recent research suggests an extract of the nut may improve the body's ability to respond to insulin and pull sugar from the blood. Cashews are also rich in magnesium, a mineral that has been associated with insulin resistance when it is lacking in the diet, as well as high blood pressure and other traits that increase the risk of heart disease, stroke, and diabetes. Cashews are lower in fat than many other popular nuts and contain little saturated fat. The fat they do contain is primarily monounsaturated oleic acid, the same fat in olive oil, which is considered heart healthy. Like other nuts, cashews provide protein and fiber, making them filling and satisfying.

Selection and Storage

Cashews are available oil-roasted and salted, but are most nutritious in their dry-roasted and unsalted form. Because of their fat content, they should be stored in an airtight container, in the refrigerator, to prevent rancidity. Always check the "sell by" date on packages of cashews to be sure they are fresh.

Tips

Cashews make wonderful nut butter and a tasty addition to salads and stir-fry dishes. As with most nuts, roasting cashews intensifies their flavor so you can use less in recipes. Enjoy cashews as a snack, but be sure to watch your portions.

NUTRIENTS PER SERVING:

Cashews, 1 ounce dry roasted without salt

Calories: 163
Protein: 4g
Total fat: 13g
Saturated fat: 2.5g
Cholesterol: 0mg
Carbohydrate: 9g
Dietary fiber: 1g
Sodium: 5mg
Potassium: 160mg
Iron: 1.7mg
Vitamin E: 0.3mg
Magnesium: 74mg
Folate: 20mcg

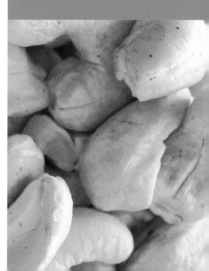

Any way you slice or shred it, cheese adds creaminess and a rich flavor to foods. Although high in fat, a little cheese goes a long way. A sprinkling of Parmesan cheese over a vegetable dish or a snack of fruit accompanied by a bit of Cheddar are indulgences that can also make nutritional sense.

Benefits

Cheese is low in carbohydrates and has very little effect on blood sugar levels. Its protein makes it a long-lasting energy source, but because it can be high in fat, it's a food to enjoy in moderation (serving size is about 1 ounce). Cheese is a concentrated source of many of the nutrients that are found in milk, including calcium, protein, phosphorus, magnesium, potassium, vitamin A, riboflavin, and vitamin B_{12}. Cheese has also been found to help protect teeth from cavity-causing bacteria.

Selection and Storage

There are more than 300 varieties of cheese, many available in various flavors and forms (sliced, cubed, shredded, spreadable, etc.). Choose reduced-fat or part-skim varieties for fewer calories and less fat. Purchase cheese by the "sell by" date and store it, tightly wrapped, in the refrigerator's cheese compartment for up to several weeks.

Tips

Cheese can be eaten alone or added to other dishes. A little cheese pairs well with fruits, vegetables, and grains, making these foods even more nutritious and delicious. Full-flavored hard cheeses, such as Parmesan or Asiago, or aromatic sharp cheeses, such as sharp Cheddar or Gorgonzola, can be used in smaller amounts to add intense flavor to dishes without a ton of excess calories.

NUTRIENTS PER SERVING:

Cheese, 1 ounce reduced-fat provolone

Calories: 77
Protein: 7g
Total fat: 5g
Saturated fat: 3g
Cholesterol: 15mg
Carbohydrate: 1g
Dietary fiber: 0g
Sodium: 245mg
Potassium: 39mg
Calcium: 212mg
Iron: 0.2mg
Vitamin A: 149 IU
Phosphorus: 139mg
Vitamin B_{12}: 0.4mcg

CINNAMON

Used for centuries as a culinary spice and for medicinal purposes, cinnamon is gaining attention as an aid for regulating blood sugar levels.

Benefits

Several studies have shown improved insulin sensitivity and blood glucose control from taking as little as ½ teaspoon of cinnamon per day. Cinnamon may also help lower blood cholesterol and triglyceride levels, which are often elevated in people with type 2 diabetes. Cinnamon contains more protective antioxidants than most other spices and many foods do. You'll find as many anti-oxidants in 1 teaspoon of cinnamon as in a full cup of pomegranate juice or ½ cup of blueberries. Cinnamon is also a good source of chromium, an essential mineral that enhances the action of insulin.

Selection and Storage

Cinnamon is available ground or as sticks, or scrolls, of dried bark. Ground cinnamon has a stronger flavor than the sticks and can stay fresh for six months; the scrolls last longer. Both should be stored in a cool, dark, dry place.

Tips

Cinnamon adds a warm, distinctive flavor to both sweet and savory dishes. It is often paired with apples and added to sweet baked goods, but also adds a pungent flavor to Middle Eastern and Asian dishes. Cinnamon is an ingredient in curry powder. Be adventurous with cin-namon—the possibilities are endless. Perk up drinks, such as coffee, tea, smoothies, or mulled wine, with ground cinnamon or sticks of cinna-mon. Sprinkle cinnamon on cereal, ice cream, pudding, or yogurt. Spice up your meats by adding cinnamon to marinades for lamb or beef.

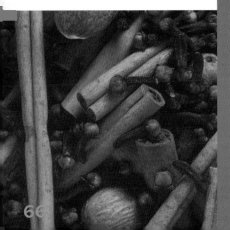

NUTRIENTS PER SERVING:

Cinnamon, 1 teaspoon ground

Calories: 6
Protein: 0g
Total fat: 0g
Saturated fat: 0g

Cholesterol: 0mg
Carbohydrate: 2g
Dietary fiber: 1g
Sodium: 0mg
Potassium: 11mg
Calcium: 26mg
Iron: 0.2mg
Vitamin A: 8 IU

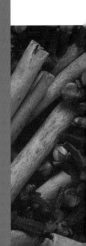

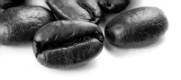

Coffee has much more to offer than a caffeine "buzz." Emerging research suggests that coffee may offer a protection against type 2 diabetes.

Benefits

A promising, but so far unexplained, scientific observation is that coffee drinkers are less likely to develop diabetes. But even for those who already have the disease, coffee may offer benefits. Both regular and decaf coffee contain minerals such as chromium and magnesium that help the body use insulin. Both minerals are rich in antioxidants, which help protect the vulnerable heart and blood vessels of a person with diabetes. Plus, plain black coffee is a great choice for anyone who is diet-conscious, as it is nearly calorie free.

Selection and Storage

You'll find myriad coffee selections at the store—from whole to ground, mild- to full-bodied, caffeinated or decaffeinated and instant to flavored. Choose the form and flavor depending on your preparation and your taste preferences. Store coffee beans or ground coffee in an airtight container in a cool, dry place. Whole beans should be used within a week or ground coffee within a few days. For long-term storage, keep coffee in the freezer.

Tips

The calorie-free beverage we should indulge in isn't always what we choose—beware of coffee drinks loaded with sugary syrups, whole milk, and whipped cream, which can add loads of calories and fat. Coffee is a wonderful flavor enhancer and adds depth to various recipes, from desserts to main dishes, including chilis, pasta sauces and marinades, or glazes for meats.

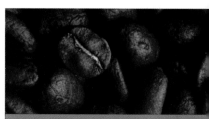

NUTRIENTS PER SERVING:

Coffee, 1 cup brewed

Calories: 2
Protein: 0g
Total Fat: 0g
Saturated fat: 0g
Cholesterol: 0mg
Carbohydrate: 0g
Dietary fiber: 0g
Sodium: 5mg
Potassium: 116mg
Magnesium: 7mg
Calcium: 5mg
Folate: 5mcg

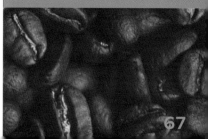

DARK CHOCOLATE

Being diabetic doesn't mean giving up chocolate! Contrary to popular belief, people with diabetes can indulge in sweets. Moderate amounts of dark chocolate can fit into your diabetes meal plan without sending your blood sugar soaring.

Benefits

Unlike other candies or sweet foods, dark chocolate has little effect on blood sugar. It contains antioxidants, essential minerals, and plant nutrients called flavanols that help protect the heart by lowering blood pressure and improving circulation. Shielding the heart from damage is particularly important for people with diabetes, since the disease increases the risk of cardiovascular disease. Still, moderation is essential, as dark chocolate is high in calories and saturated fat. To get the most benefit without overdoing calories, enjoy only 1 or 2 ounces per week.

Selection and Storage

Dark chocolate is available in varying levels of "darkness," depending on the percentage of cocoa. For example, 60 percent cocoa content means that 40 percent of the product is made up of sugar, vanilla, and other ingredients. The higher the percentage of cocoa, the less sweet and more bitter it will taste. Dark chocolate includes semisweet and bittersweet varieties. Store dark chocolate tightly wrapped in a cool, dry place. Warmer temperatures will cause grayish streaks and blotches, which do not affect flavor. Under ideal conditions, dark chocolate can be stored for years without losing quality.

Tips

Dark chocolate is best enjoyed on its own. It can also be used in baking, in a wide variety of desserts or simply as a garnish for a low-calorie dessert.

NUTRIENTS PER SERVING:

Dark chocolate, 1 ounce

Calories: 154
Protein: 1g
Total fat: 9g
Saturated fat: 5g
Cholesterol: 2mg
Carbohydrate: 17g

Dietary fiber: 2g
Sodium: 6mg
Potassium: 160mg
Calcium: 16mg
Iron: 2.3mg
Magnesium: 43mg
Copper: 0.3mg
Phosphorus: 60mg

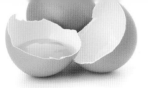

EGGS

For years, eggs have been shed in a negative light. Yet the incredible egg is quite beneficial. Eating eggs is a great way to start your day, as they are rich in protein and many nutrients.

Benefits

Even though eggs are high in cholesterol, research indicates they can be a healthy addition to a diabetes meal plan. Eggs offer 13 essential vitamins and minerals, high-quality protein, healthy unsaturated fats, and protective antioxidants, all for about 75 calories per egg. Enjoying eggs at breakfast has been shown to help control both hunger and blood sugar levels. But what about all that cholesterol? It turns out the saturated fat in the foods we eat, far more than the cholesterol content, is what jacks up cholesterol levels. And eggs are actually rather low in saturated fats. Keep in mind that pairing eggs with bacon and sausage—foods loaded with saturated fat—will not favor your cholesterol levels.

Selection and Storage

Choose eggs that are clean and not cracked, and always check the "sell by" date for freshness. Brown eggs and those labeled as "farm-laid" or "free-range" are no more nutritious. However, eggs from hens fed a diet rich in omega-3 fatty acids will contain more of this healthy fat. Store eggs in the carton in the main part of the refrigerator, and use within three weeks.

Tips

From scrambled eggs to egg soufflé, eggs are a versatile food on their own. They also serve as an essential ingredient in recipes—helping baked goods to rise, binding ingredients in casseroles, thickening custards and sauces, and emulsifying mayonnaise and salad dressings, to name a few.

NUTRIENTS PER SERVING:

Egg, 1 large boiled

Calories: 78
Protein: 6g
Total fat: 5g
Saturated fat: 2g
Cholesterol: 186mg
Carbohydrate: <1g
Dietary fiber: 0g
Sodium: 60mg
Potassium: 65mg
Calcium: 25mg
Iron: 0.6mg
Vitamin A: 260 IU
Vitamin D: 44 IU
Choline: 113mg

MUSHROOMS

Mushrooms can be enjoyed in countless ways, but their hearty texture makes them best enjoyed as a low-calorie meat substitute.

Benefits

Mushrooms are essentially a "free food" in a diabetic diet, as they are very low in calories and carbohydrates. They are also virtually sodium-free and provide hefty amounts of potassium, which benefits the many people with diabetes who also have high blood pressure. What makes mushrooms stand out is that they are the only source of vitamin D found in the produce aisle. Many varieties of mushrooms are also rich in selenium, an antioxidant mineral with anticancer properties.

Selection and Storage

All supermarkets stock the white button mushroom, and many have expanded their selection to include other varieties such as shiitake, chanterelle, enoki, morel, oyster, Portobello, and the often dried Chinese wood-ear. Mushrooms like cool, humid, circulating air and need to be stored in a paper bag or ventilated container in your refrigerator, but not in the crisper drawer. Mushrooms last only a couple of days, but can still be used to impart flavor in cooking after they've turned brown.

Tips

To clean, use a mushroom brush or wipe mushrooms with a damp cloth. Don't cut mushrooms until you're ready to use them. Mushrooms cook quickly. They'll absorb oil in cooking, so it's best to sauté mushrooms in broth or wine. Try going meatless sometimes. Portobello mushrooms are good for grilling and can take the place of meat in many dishes, including burgers and meat loaves.

NUTRIENTS PER SERVING:

Mushrooms,
½ cup cooked

Calories: 22
Protein: 2g
Total fat: 1g
Saturated fat: 0g
Cholesterol: 0mg
Carbohydrate: 4g
Dietary fiber: 2g
Sodium: 0mg
Potassium: 278mg
Calcium: 5mg
Iron: 1.4mg
Vitamin D: 16.4 IU
Selenium: 9mcg
Niacin: 3.5mg
Riboflavin: 0.2mg

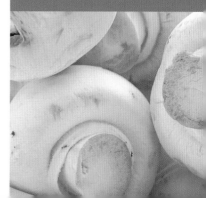

ORANGES

In addition to providing insoluble fiber to help with blood sugar control, oranges pack nutrients that battle diabetes complications. Plus, they have a sweet, tart flavor that makes them wonderful substitutes for high-calorie snacks and desserts.

Benefits

This juicy fruit is best known for providing vitamin C to help prevent you from getting sick, but for people with diabetes, the benefits go way beyond this. One orange provides 130 percent of the daily requirement for vitamin C, which helps control infections, maintain healthy teeth and gums, and protect small blood vessels. As an antioxidant, vitamin C works with the folate and potassium found in oranges to slow the development of coronary heart disease. Vitamin C and the orange-related phytochemical beta-carotene also support eye health and lower the risk of sight-stealing cataracts.

Selection and Storage

Oranges are one of the few fruits abundant in winter. California navels are the most popular oranges for eating on their own. The Valencias, produced in Florida, are the premier juice-producing oranges. Mandarin oranges are small and sweet with thin skins and easily sectioned segments and are also available canned. For all varieties, select firm fruit heavy for its size, indicating juiciness.

Green color and blemishes are fine. Refrigerated, most varieties, except mandarins, will keep for two weeks. Orange juice is available fresh squeezed or from concentrate. Just be sure it is 100 percent juice with no added sugar.

Tips

For fruit salads or eating out of hand, choose seedless oranges. Or top your favorite spinach salad with some orange segments. Try using fresh orange juice to make marinades or nonfat sauces and dressings.

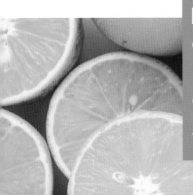

NUTRIENTS PER SERVING:

Orange (navel), 1 medium

Calories: 69
Protein: 1g
Total fat: 0g

Saturated fat: 0g
Cholesterol: 0mg
Carbohydrate: 18g
Dietary fiber: 3g
Sodium: 0mg
Potassium: 230mg

Calcium: 60mg
Iron: 0.2mg
Vitamin A: 346 IU
Vitamin C: 83mg
Folate: 48mcg

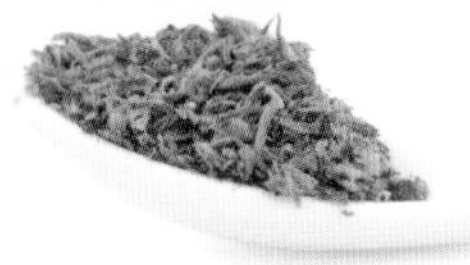

OREGANO

Skip harmful seasonings and sauces and sprinkle food with oregano to impart wonderful flavor. Of all the herbs, oregano has one of the highest antioxidant levels.

Benefits

Beyond its role as a healthy flavor enhancer, oregano carries antioxidant nutrients that may give it even greater disease-fighting potential. Research into oregano's possible benefits is only in preliminary stages but suggests the herb may help with blood-sugar control as well as have positive effects on heart health and the integrity of blood vessels. Additionally, the lutein and zeaxanthin found in oregano may help prevent cataracts and certain other eye diseases.

Selection and Storage

Fresh oregano is often available in supermarkets. Choose bright green, fresh-looking bunches with no sign of wilting or yellowing. Refrigerate in a plastic bag for up to three days. Dried oregano is available in both crumbled and ground forms. It should be stored in a cool, dark place. For the best flavor and to get the maximum nutritional benefits, use dried oregano within six months.

Tips

Oregano has an aromatic scent and robust taste. It goes extremely well with tomato-based dishes, such as marinara sauce, tomato soup, and pizza. It also enhances cheese and egg dishes and can be used to add flavor to stews, soups, and chili. Oregano can be combined with other herbs and garlic to create a rub marinade for meats. Fresh oregano is best used at the end of cooking or sprinkled on foods just before eating, whereas dried oregano can be added during cooking.

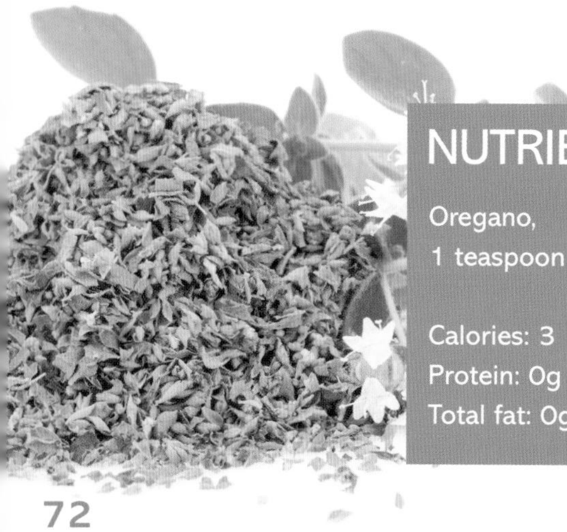

NUTRIENTS PER SERVING:

Oregano, 1 teaspoon dried

Calories: 3
Protein: 0g
Total fat: 0g

Saturated fat: 0g
Cholesterol: 0mg
Carbohydrate: <1g
Dietary fiber: 0.5g
Sodium: 0mg

Potassium: 13mg
Calcium: 16mg
Iron: 0.4mg
Vitamin A: 17 IU
Folate: 2mcg

PASTA

This comfort food is no longer banned from a diabetic diet. Whole wheat and whole grain pastas are a tasty way to enjoy this favorite fare without worrying about your blood sugar.

Benefits

Whole grain and whole wheat pastas are naturally rich in fiber, which slows the absorption of sugar, and in minerals, such as magnesium, that increase the body's sensitivity to insulin. This makes whole wheat or whole grain pasta a must, as these beneficial ingredients are typically lost or significantly reduced when grains are refined. Additionally, newer varieties of healthy pastas, including products with added fiber, are especially helpful for diabetic diets.

Selection and Storage

To simplify your pasta choices, look for products labeled as whole wheat or whole grain. These are widely available in all supermarkets and convenience stores. Whole wheat pasta is darker in color and tends to have a chewier texture than white varieties. Whole grain pasta is made with a mix of nutrient-rich ingredients, including legumes, oats, barley, flax, and egg whites. Whole wheat and whole grain pastas cook about the same as white—just follow package instructions to be sure. Dried pasta will keep in your cupboard for several months.

Tips

Pasta is best cooked until al dente—tender yet chewy. Drain immediately and do not rinse. To prevent sticking, immediately toss with a low-fat vegetable sauce or olive oil. For a meatless meal, toss some whole wheat pasta with your favorite beans and vegetables, drizzle with olive oil, and add a squeeze of lemon and some fresh herbs.

NUTRIENTS PER SERVING:

Pasta (whole wheat), ½ cup cooked

Calories: 87
Protein: 3.5g
Total fat: 0g
Saturated fat: 0g
Cholesterol: 0mg
Carbohydrate: 19g
Dietary fiber: 3g
Sodium: 0mg
Potassium: 30mg
Calcium: 10mg
Iron: 0.7mg
Vitamin A: 2 IU
Folate: 4mcg

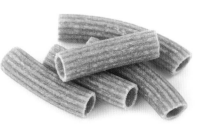

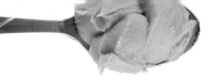

PEANUT BUTTER

Because it is rich in protein, peanut butter is great in any diet. Peanut butter provides long-lasting energy and essential heart-protective nutrients with little effect on blood sugar.

Benefits

The combination of protein, fiber, and fat found in peanut butter means it digests more slowly and provides fuel over time without causing blood sugar spikes. Peanut butter also has a vast amount of benefits on heart health. Peanut butter is rich in monounsaturated fats, which help lower LDL (bad) cholesterol; niacin, which helps raise HDL (good) cholesterol levels; and potassium for blood pressure control. Additionally, peanut butter contains a high amount of magnesium, a mineral that is often found in low levels in people with diabetes.

Selection and Storage

Peanut butter is available many varieties: creamy or chunky, natural or blended, unsalted, reduced-fat, reduced-sodium, and re-duced-sugar. Natural peanut butter is unprocessed and the oil may separate out. Simply stir to combine and refrigerate, where it will remain fresh about six months. To make your own peanut butter, place shelled peanuts in the food processor and grind until you have achieved the desired consistency. Homemade peanut butter keeps about three months in the refrigerator. When buying from the store, look for peanut butters with little or no added sugar.

Tips

Rather than your typical PB&J, try a peanut butter and banana or peanut butter and honey sandwich. But peanut butter has many uses besides sandwiches. Enjoy it for a snack spread on apple wedges, pears, crackers, or toast. Pay attention to portion sizes—a little peanut butter goes a long way.

NUTRIENTS PER SERVING:

Peanut butter, 2 tablespoons unsalted (low sodium)
Calories: 188
Protein: 8g
Total fat: 16g
Saturated fat: 3g
Monounsaturated fat: 8g
Polyunsaturated fat: 4g
Cholesterol: 0mg
Carbohydrate: 6g
Dietary fiber: 2g
Sodium: 5mg
Potassium: 208mg
Magnesium: 49mg
Phosphorus: 115mg
Calcium: 14mg
Iron: 1mg
Folate: 41mcg
Niacin: 4mg
Vitamin B$_6$: 0.2mg
Vitamin E: 3mg

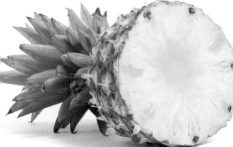

PINEAPPLE

Pineapple gets high scores for its exceptionally sweet and tart taste and health-protective nutrients. It's a great way to satisfy your sweet tooth, too.

Benefits

Pineapple provides more than a third of the daily recommended allowance of vitamin C, an antioxidant that helps with immune health. This is important for people with diabetes because they a have a higher risk of infection. Vitamin C is also a powerful antioxidant that helps protect against diabetes-related heart disease. Pineapple offers heart-protective folate and potassium, as well, which are needed for healthy blood pressure.

Selection and Storage

When choosing pineapple, let your nose be your guide. A ripe pineapple gives off a sweet aroma from its base. Color is not a reliable indicator; ripe pineapples vary in color by variety. Choose a large pineapple that feels heavy for its size, indicating juiciness and a lot of pulp. A ripe pineapple yields slightly when pressed. Once a pineapple is picked, it will not ripen further. Canned pineapple is available; be sure to select varieties packed in juice or water, not syrup.

Tips

Preparing a pineapple is not as scary it looks. Cut off the bottom and top, then peel the outside using a sharp knife. Remove any remaining "eyes." Cut into quarters and remove the core from each quarter and cut into slices. Add pineapple to a fruit smoothie or to top low-fat yogurt. Use pineapple in fruit salad or make fruit kabobs for a unique dessert. Pineapple works well when grilled. Try it alone for dessert or on a kabob with your favorite meat.

NUTRIENTS PER SERVING:

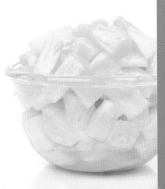

Pineapple,
½ cup raw

Calories: 41
Protein: 1g
Total fat: 0g

Saturated fat: 0g
Cholesterol: 0mg
Carbohydrate: 11g
Dietary fiber: 1g
Sodium: 0mg
Potassium: 90mg

Calcium: 11mg
Iron: 0.2mg
Manganese: 0.8mg
Vitamin C: 39mg
Folate: 15mcg

PISTACHIOS

Compared to other popular nuts, pistachios are among the highest in protein and fiber and also one of the lowest in calories and fat. And they offer loads of key nutrients, as well.

Benefits

Pistachios are useful for the many people with diabetes who also have heart disease. These yummy green nuts are full of phytosterols, natural compounds that compete with cholesterol for absorption by the body, helping reduce blood cholesterol levels. They also contain arginine, an amino acid that helps improve circulation. Pistachios are rich in monounsaturated fats, the same heart-healthy fats found in olive oil. And they provide a hefty amount of resveratrol, a phytonutrient (also found in wine) that may play a role in fighting heart disease and cancer. Additionally, pistachios offer noteworthy amounts of potassium, magnesium, copper, vitamin B_6, and vitamin E.

Selection and Storage

Pistachios are increasingly available shelled but are more expensive than the commonly found unshelled forms. They are available either raw or roasted, and salted or unsalted. When buying unshelled pistachios, the shells should be partly opened, which not only makes it easier to remove the nut, but also indicates that the nut is mature and ready to be eaten. Store pistachios in an airtight container in the refrigerator or freezer for up to one year.

Tips

Pistachios work well in savory or sweet dishes. They can be toasted and added to vegetable or rice dishes. Or sprinkle a handful of chopped pistachios on breakfast cereal or salads for an extra crunch. Swap them out with walnuts that are traditionally used in baking. Incorporate them into muffins, cakes, or cookies.

NUTRIENTS PER SERVING:

Pistachios, 1 ounce dry roasted without salt

Calories: 161
Protein: 6g
Total fat: 13g
Saturated fat: 1.5g
Cholesterol: 0mg
Carbohydrate: 8g
Dietary fiber: 3g
Sodium: 0mg
Potassium: 285mg
Calcium: 30mg
Iron: 1.1mg
Vitamin A: 73 IU
Vitamin C: 1mg
Folate: 14mcg
Magnesium: 31mg
Vitamin E: 0.7mg

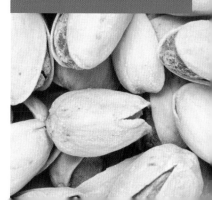

POPCORN

Popcorn is a surprising snack food that people with diabetes can indulge in. Like other whole grain sources of carbohydrate, air-popped and unprocessed popcorn is a good source of fiber and nutrients.

Benefits

Plain popcorn is a delicious snack that's naturally low in calories and fat. Plus, you can have a large volume for a small amount of calories. Because it's made from corn, a whole grain, popcorn doesn't impact blood sugar levels as much as many other snack foods. Popcorn has a lower glycemic load than raisins, rice cakes, or potato chips. Air-popped popcorn without added butter or oil is a good source of potassium, magnesium, and phosphorus.

Selection and Storage

Popcorn is available in the snack food aisle in various flavors and forms. Buy popcorn kernels to pop yourself on the stovetop or in an air popper, or look for low-fat microwave popcorn. Avoid the heavily salted and buttery varieties of popcorn. Choose low-fat varieties of popcorn without added fats, sugars, and salts.

Tips

Rather than dousing your popcorn in butter and salt, experiment with healthier alternatives that add flavor, not guilt. Try adding garlic powder rather than salt. If you love kettle corn, try sprinkling ground cinnamon and a sugar substitute for sweet snack.

NUTRIENTS PER SERVING:

Popcorn, 2 cups air-popped without added butter or oil

Calories: 62	Dietary fiber: 2g
Protein: 2g	Calcium: 1mg
Total fat: 1g	Potassium: 53mg
Saturated fat: 0g	Sodium: 1mg
Cholesterol: 0mg	Magnesium: 23mg
Carbohydrate: 12g	Phosphorus: 57mg

PORK TENDERLOIN

Chicken no longer has to be the center of your plate. Pork tenderloin is lean and rich in plenty of nutrients, making it a great substitute for the poultry you may be getting sick of.

Benefits

Pork tenderloin is comparable to skinless chicken breast in calories, total fat, and saturated fat. It is also lower in cholesterol, so it's a good fit for a heart healthy diabetes diet. Its high quality protein leaves you feeling satisfied, which will help in any weight-loss efforts. Pork tenderloin also provides more than 20 percent of your daily requirements for many B vitamins, including thiamin, niacin, riboflavin, vitamin B$_6$, and the mineral phosphorus.

This is significant since the body needs B vitamins to turn food into energy.

Selection and Storage

Pork tenderloin is long and thin and easy to find in the fresh meat section of the supermarket. About 4 ounces raw will yield a 3-ounce cooked serving. Prepackaged fresh pork tenderloin can be stored in the refrigerator for up to four days. Well-wrapped, it can be stored in the freezer for up to six months.

Tips

Pork tenderloin makes an elegant entrée for a dinner party but also can easily be roasted or grilled for a quick meal. It has a mild flavor, so it's best when prepared with an added spice rub, marinade, stuffing, or flavorful sauce. To keep the tenderloin juicy, be careful not to overcook it. A meat thermometer inserted into the thickest part of the meat should reach a temperature of 160°F for medium doneness.

NUTRIENTS PER SERVING:

Pork tenderloin,
3 ounces roasted

Calories: 125
Protein: 22g
Total fat: 3.5g
Saturated fat: 1g
Cholesterol: 62mg
Carbohydrate: <1g

Dietary fiber: 0g
Sodium: 50mg
Potassium: 355mg
Thiamin: 0.8mg
Riboflavin: 0.3mg
Niacin: 6.3mg
Vitamin B$_6$: 0.6mg
Phosphorus: 225mg

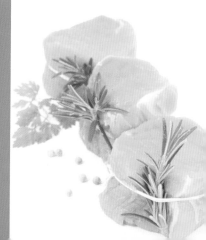

RYE

Move over, wheat! Foods made from rye may be less common, but their hearty flavor and numerous health benefits make them worth including in your meal plan.

Benefits

Like other whole grains, rye products—such as traditional rye bread and pumpernickel—are rich in fiber that helps keep blood sugar from skyrocketing following a meal. Compared to regular wheat bread, rye bread has also been shown to trigger less of an insulin response, so blood sugar is less likely to plunge, too. And as an added bonus, rye foods keep you feeling satisfied longer, making it easier to manage your appetite between meals, which may help you lose those extra pounds.

Selection and Storage

Rye grains may be available whole, cracked, or rolled, but are generally ground into flour. Light rye flour has most of the bran (fiber) removed, while dark rye flour retains most of the bran and germ, so it has more fiber and nu-trients. Store rye grains in an airtight container in a cool, dry, dark place, where they will keep for several months. Rye bread is available in the bread section of the supermarket. Read labels carefully, as what is labeled "rye bread" is sometimes wheat bread with caramel coloring.

Tips

Rye bread is generally more compact and dense than wheat bread, so it works well for toasting or for sandwiches with hearty and moist fillings. Rye bread pairs well with corned beef. For a tasty snack or appetizer, make Reuben bites. Bake party-size rye bread slices in a 400°F oven for 5 minutes. Spread fat-free Thousand Island dressing on the mini bread slices. Top with turkey pastrami and shredded reduced-fat Swiss cheese. Bake for another 5 minutes.

Top with alfalfa sprouts and serve immediately.

NUTRIENTS PER SERVING:

Rye bread, 1 slice

Calories: 83
Protein: 3g
Total fat: 1g
Saturated fat: 0g
Cholesterol: 0mg
Carbohydrate: 15g
Dietary fiber: 2g
Sodium: 211mg
Potassium: 53mg
Calcium: 23mg
Iron: 0.9mg
Thiamin: 0.14mg
Riboflavin: 0.1mg
Folate: 35mcg

SHRIMP

Shrimp is a lean protein source that can be easily added to a diabetic meal. Although high in cholesterol, shrimp are naturally low in total fat and saturated fat, making them a good choice for anyone on a low-fat diet.

Benefits

Shrimp are lean, high in protein, and rich in nutrients. They supply heart-healthy omega-3 fat, which is associated with a lower risk of heart disease, certain cancers, and age-related eye diseases. Research also suggests omega-3s are important to cognitive function and may help lower elevated blood pressure and reduce joint inflammation in arthritis. Although shrimp are rich in omega-3s, they are low in total fat compared to most complete protein sources. And they're very low in cholesterol-raising saturated fat. Shrimp also contain more heart-protective vitamin B_{12} and fewer calories, ounce for ounce, than other sources of animal protein.

Selection and Storage

Buy shrimp from a trusted source with a good reputation for having fresh seafood. Frozen shrimp keep for several weeks in the freezer. Fresh shrimp should be eaten within a day or two of purchase. Select fresh shrimp with firm bodies still attached to their shells and no black spots. Frozen shrimp should be tightly wrapped and stored in the freezer for up to one month.

Tips

Shrimp can be served as a main course or added to other dishes, such as soups, salads, stews, and stir-fries. Shrimp can be cooked with or without shells—follow recipe instructions. Frozen shrimp should be thawed in the refrigerator before cooking. To devein shrimp (optional), make a shallow cut along the rounded side and use the tip of a knife or your fingers to remove the black, string-like vein.

NUTRIENTS PER SERVING:

Shrimp, 3 ounces cooked

Calories: 101
Protein: 19g
Total fat: 2g
Saturated fat: 0g
Cholesterol: 179mg
Carbohydrate: 1g
Dietary fiber: 0g
Sodium: 805mg
Potassium: 145mg
Calcium: 77mg
Iron: 0.3mg
Magnesium: 31mg
Copper: 0.2mg
Vitamin B_{12}: 1.4mcg

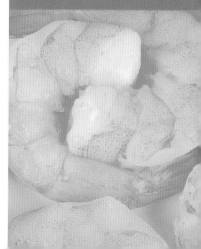

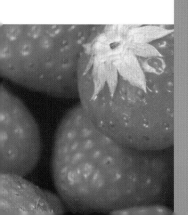

STRAWBERRIES

Finding something to satisfy a sweet tooth can seem difficult for diabetics. But juicy strawberries make a great low-calorie, fiber-filled sweet that can stand in for high-calorie desserts and snacks.

Benefits

Strawberries are rich in a variety of phytonutrients that protect the heart and assist in blood sugar control. Recent research found that the polyphenols in strawberries may have the ability to blunt a rise in blood sugar levels after consuming table sugar. Eating strawberries several times a week also appears to be associated with a lower risk of type 2 diabetes. Strawberries are an exceptional source of vitamin C; they contain more than oranges and grapefruit.

Selection and Storage

Look for plump strawberries that are ruby red, evenly colored, and have green, leafy tops. Avoid those that appear mushy or bruised. Bigger does not equal better. Smaller strawberries tend to be the sweetest. Avoid strawberries in containers with juice stains or berries packed tightly with plastic wrap. Strawberries spoil quickly; it's best to serve them within a couple days of purchasing.

Tips

Though they are delicious on their own, strawberries can perk up several types of dishes. Add some sliced strawberries to your morning bowl of cereal or yogurt, to a spinach salad, or serve with pudding. You can add overripe strawberries to smoothies or fruit drinks or create a sauce for fruit salads or desserts. Add a splash of balsamic vinegar to bring out the sweet flavor of strawberries.

NUTRIENTS PER SERVING:

Strawberries, 1 cup halved raw

Calories: 49
Protein: 1g
Total fat: 0g
Saturated fat: 0g
Cholesterol: 0mg
Carbohydrate: 12g

Dietary fiber: 3g
Sodium: 0mg
Potassium: 235mg
Calcium: 24mg
Iron: 0.6mg
Vitamin A: 18 IU
Vitamin C: 89mg
Folate: 36mcg

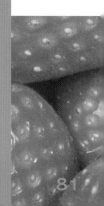

SWEET POTATOES

This tasty tuber shouldn't only be eaten at Thanksgiving. Rich in flavor and nutrients, sweet potatoes have much to offer in a diabetic diet.

Benefits

The carotenoids in sweet potatoes appear to help stabilize blood sugar levels due to their ability to lower insulin resistance by making cells more responsive to the hormone. These effects not only aid in disease management, but also make it easier to drop the excess pounds, which tend to aggravate the disease. Sweet potatoes also offer fiber to keep you full for hours. Furthermore, the hefty nutrient profile can help protect your heart and the rest of your body from damage and complications related to diabetes. For example, they supply infection-fighting vitamin C and blood pressure-lowering potassium.

Selection and Storage

Though often called a yam, a sweet potato is a different vegetable. Look for sweet potatoes that are small to medium in size with smooth, unbruised skin. Though sweet potatoes look rather tough and hard, they're actually quite fragile and spoil easily. Any cut or bruise on the surface quickly spreads, ruining the whole potato. Store potatoes at room temperature, as refrigeration will speed up deterioration.

Tips

To prepare sweet potatoes, boil unpeeled potatoes, or bake or microwave them whole. Leaving the peel intact prevents excessive loss of precious nutrients and locks in its natural sweetness. Try sweet potatoes mashed, roasted, or in a soufflé. Use them to add moisture, flavor, and a boon of nutrients to quick breads or muffins.

NUTRIENTS PER SERVING:

Sweet potatoes, ½ cup baked

Calories: 90
Protein: 2g
Total fat: 0g
Saturated fat: 0g
Cholesterol: 0mg
Carbohydrate: 21g
Dietary fiber: 3.5g
Sodium: 35mg
Potassium: 475mg
Calcium: 38mg
Iron: 0.7mg
Vitamin A: 19,218 IU
Vitamin C: 20mg
Folate: 6mcg

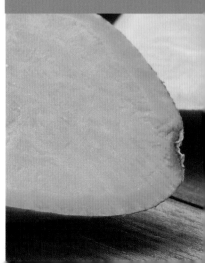

WALNUTS

Compared to other nuts, walnuts provide the most omega-3 fats. Eating a handful of them daily is a delicious way to battle diabetes.

Benefits

Eaten in moderation, walnuts are especially helpful for people with type 2 diabetes. They've been shown to reduce common dangerous characteristics of the disease, including insulin resistance, excess body weight, and increased risk of heart disease. Walnuts provide a hefty amount of alpha-linolenic acid, the plant-based source of omega-3 fats that helps prevent blood clotting, reduce inflammation, and lower triglyceride levels in the blood. Walnuts also supply protein and soluble fiber, a combination of nutrients that helps to satisfy hunger, lower cholesterol, and smooth out blood sugar fluctuations.

Selection and Storage

Walnuts are most often available shelled but can also be purchased in the shell. Look for walnut shells without cracks or stains. Shelled walnuts are available whole, chopped, or ground and should be crisp rather than limp or rubbery. Check the freshness date before buying them. Store shelled walnuts in the refrigerator to prevent rancidity. In the shell, walnuts can be stored in a cool, dry place for up to a year.

Tips

Walnuts can be enjoyed out of hand or chopped and added to many different foods. Roasting walnuts brings out the flavor. You can add them to homemade granola or use them to top oatmeal, cereal, or yogurt. They are a wonderful addition to salads and vegetable dishes, as well. And the uses in muffins, pancakes, quick breads, and cookies are endless.

NUTRIENTS PER SERVING:

Walnuts, 1 ounce dry roasted without salt

Calories: 185
Protein: 4g
Total fat: 18.5g
Saturated fat: 1.5g
Cholesterol: 0mg
Carbohydrate: 4g

Dietary fiber: 2g
Sodium: 0mg
Potassium: 125mg
Calcium: 28mg
Iron: 0.8mg
Folate: 28mcg
Magnesium: 45mg
Vitamin E: 0.2 mg

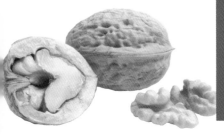

WHEAT BRAN

Literally bursting with fiber, wheat bran—the hard outer shell of the wheat kernel—offers an easy way to boost the fiber in almost anything you eat.

Benefits

Wheat bran is a great tool for increasing fiber intake as it can easily be incorporated into numerous foods. And for people with diabetes, eating a fiber-rich diet, filled with whole grains, fruits, and vegetables, is essential in keeping blood sugar in a healthier range. Fiber-rich foods play an important role in weight loss, too, which is important for those with diabetes who need to lose weight to improve their condition. Wheat bran also contributes heart-protective nutrients, such as niacin, which boosts HDL (good) cholesterol levels, and potassium and magnesium, which help lower blood pressure.

Selection and Storage

Wheat bran is usually available in bulk bins in the natural foods section of the supermarket, or it may be found with grains or cereals. Wheat bran is best stored in airtight containers in the refrigerator for prolonged shelf life.

Tips

Wheat bran can be added to many foods to boost fiber content. Sprinkle it over hot or cold cereals or on yogurt or applesauce. Add wheat bran to recipes for breads, cookies, muffins, and pancakes. It can easily be added to ground meat dishes, such as meat loaves, burgers, or casseroles. Toasting wheat bran gives is an especially nutty flavor and crunchy texture.

NUTRIENTS PER SERVING:

Wheat bran, ½ cup

Calories: 63
Protein: 5g
Total fat: 1g
Saturated fat: 0g
Cholesterol: 0mg
Carbohydrate: 19g
Dietary fiber: 12g
Sodium: 0mg
Potassium: 345mg
Magnesium: 177mg
Iron: 3.1mg
Zinc: 2.1mg
Niacin: 3.9mg
Vitamin B_6: 0.4mg

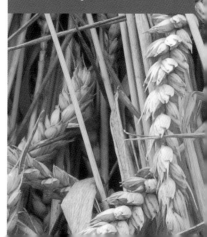

YOGURT

Yogurt has a hefty nutrient profile and can be enjoyed in several ways, making it an ally in diabetes management.

Benefits

Yogurt is great for people with diabetes. It's a nutrient-rich substitute for higher-calorie sugary desserts and provides satisfying protein to help battle hunger and even out blood sugar between meals and snacks. The protein content in yogurt allows it to be used easily in meals as a substitute for high-fat meats. And the live active bacteria cultures found in most yogurt help with digestive health by suppressing the growth of harmful bacteria in the intestinal tract. These beneficial bacteria promote immune health, too. Stronger immune function may help counter the increased vulnerability to infections that comes with diabetes.

Selection and Storage

To keep fat and calories low, look for low-fat or nonfat yogurt. The addition of fruit or sweeteners adds calories, so look for plain varieties and add your own flavorings. Some yogurt products are sweetened with noncaloric sweeteners. Check for a "sell by" date on the yogurt carton. It will keep for up to ten days past that date.

Tips

Yogurt makes a great portable meal or snack on its own, but it has several other great uses. Yogurt makes a wonderful base for smoothies when blended with fresh fruit and juice. Or top your morning bowl of cereal with yogurt instead of milk. Yogurt works as a great substitute in recipes that call for high-fat ingredients like cream or sour cream, such as tuna or chicken salad recipes. And yogurt is especially well suited as a base for dips and salad dressings.

NUTRIENTS PER SERVING:

Yogurt, 1 cup plain low-fat

Calories: 154	Sodium: 170mg
Protein: 13g	Potassium: 575mg
Total fat: 4g	Calcium: 448mg
Saturated fat: 2.5g	Iron: 0.2mg
Cholesterol: 15mg	Vitamin A: 125 IU
Carbohydrate: 17g	Vitamin C: 2mg
Dietary fiber: 0g	Folate: 27mcg

EXERCISING

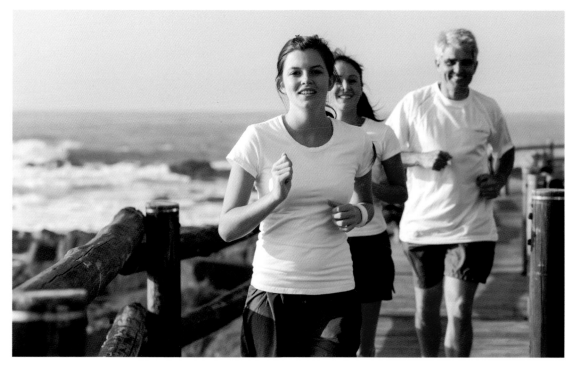

You may not think of a brisk walk, a game of tennis, or an hour spent cleaning your house as medicine for treating your diabetes, but it is. Regular exercise carries a lot of benefits for people with diabetes. It's a potent tool for lowering blood sugar because it improves the way insulin works. In fact, by incorporating regular exercise into their lives, many people with type 2 diabetes can increase their insulin sensitivity enough that they no longer need insulin injections or diabetes pills. For folks who have been diagnosed with prediabetes, it is even possible to prevent the full-blown disease through physical activity.

Not only that, but physical activity is a proven way to combat conditions that often affect people with diabetes: heart disease, high blood pressure, infection, elevated cholesterol, depression, and increased stress. It burns extra calories—an important added benefit for those who need to lose weight. Physical activity also produces chemical messengers called endorphins that help relieve anxiety and pain. In short, exercise is one of the most effective tools you can use to combat diabetes.

Incorporating Activity

This doesn't mean you should run out and get a gym membership—especially if you wouldn't use it. Instead, take steps to incorporate more movement in your daily life. Especially if you've been a couch potato of late, those first steps toward becoming more active don't even have to look like exercise in the traditional sense.

Being physically active every day is as much a state of mind as it is a state of being. It means taking every opportunity you can to move more. For many people with blood sugar problems, the simple act of walking more may be enough to start setting things right. To increase motivation, a wearable fitness tracker or pedometer can work wonders. These small devices can track the number of times your hips shift position each day. They can count every time you get up, sit down, turn, jump, and step. They also remind you that movement is good. Research has shown that people who wear pedometers and check them periodically throughout the day are motivated to walk and move more.

Here are some simple ways to incorporate movement into your daily life:

- Use a cordless or mobile phone. Get in the habit of walking while you talk.

- When you go shopping, park farther away from the store's entrance.

- Take the stairs instead of elevators and escalators, particularly when going only one or two levels.

- At airports, if you're using one of the moving walkways, walk instead of standing still.

- At work, if you need to talk to a colleague on the other side of the building, walk instead of calling or e-mailing.

- If you have a dog, volunteer to be the person who walks it.

- Don't just sit in front of the TV. Hide the TV remote and get up to change channels. Buy a treadmill, stair-stepper, or small elliptical machine, and use it while you watch TV.

- Do your own yard work.

- Do your own housework.

Developing an Exercise Routine

Once you begin adding more movement into your daily routine, the next step—establishing an exercise routine—will come much easier. Since you are looking to incorporate exercise into your daily routine, the activity you choose should also be something that you enjoy, that you have easy access to, and that is safe and reasonable for you to perform given your current health, abilities, and schedule.

Your selection will also need a thumbs-up from your doctor, especially if you haven't been active recently.

Besides deciding on a type of exercise, you also need to consider when you will exercise, how often, for how long, and how intensely. If you have an exercise physiologist on your diabetes care team, you can work together to devise an effective, challenging, and safe exercise program that evolves as your fitness increases.

Guidelines for Activity

- See your physician for a complete medical exam before adopting a new workout regimen.

- Choose activities that fit your physical condition, lifestyle, and tastes. Many people who have not been physically active for a while find that easy, low-impact activities such as walking and swimming are perfect.

- Make sure that whatever activities you choose are enjoyable for you. That increases the likelihood that you'll stick with it.

- Vary your activities so you don't get bored and fall prey to excuses. Choose some activities that can be done indoors in case of bad weather. Select some activities that can fit into a busy schedule.

- Don't skimp on exercise gear and equipment. Good-quality equipment pays for itself in the form of better protection against injuries. That's especially true for

BENEFITS OF BEING MORE ACTIVE

- Lower blood glucose
- Lower blood pressure
- Lower blood fats
- Better cardiovascular (heart and lung) fitness
- Weight loss and/or maintenance
- Improved sense of well-being

footwear. And always wear socks to keep your feet dry.

- Warm up and cool down. Begin each exercise session with a five- to ten-minute period of low-intensity activity and gentle stretching. This prepares your heart for increased activity. It also gives your muscles and joints a little time to get warm and loose. End your workouts with ten minutes of cool-down and more gentle stretching.

- Increase the amount of physical activity you do and its intensity slowly and build up gradually.

- Stay hydrated. Drink plenty of water before, during, and after exercise. Dehydration can spoil a good workout.

- Identify yourself. Just to be safe, always wear a bracelet, necklace, or shoe tag identifying yourself as a person with diabetes when you work out.

One thing is clear: The benefits of getting physical are well worth the effort. So work with your diabetes care team to create a personalized exercise program that suits your needs.

In this chapter, you'll find step-by-step instructions and accompanying photographs for:

- cardiovascular exercises to keep your heart and lungs healthy

- strength-training exercises to challenge your muscles

- exercises that use a fitness ball for balance and variety

- yoga exercises for flexibility

LOW-IMPACT ACTIVITIES

- Swimming
- Cycling
- Power walking
- Hiking
- Rowing
- Stair climbing
- Using an elliptical trainer
- Dancing
- Water aerobics

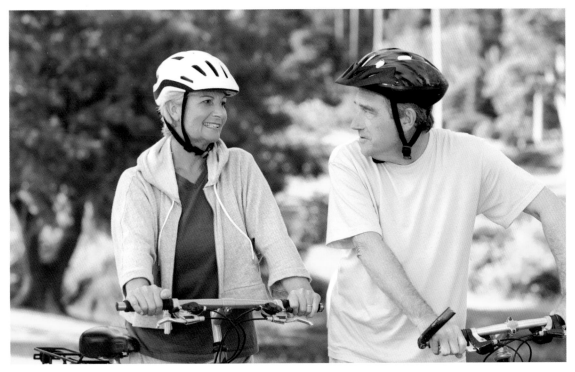

A FEW WORDS OF CAUTION

Although all diabetes patients should strive to be physically active, some forms of exercise require extra precautions (or may be too risky, period) for people who have any of the following complications.

AUTONOMIC NEUROPATHY

Patients who have this form of nerve damage may not be able to detect symptoms such as sweating and rapid heart rate that signal the onset of exercise-induced hypoglycemia. They also have a high risk for orthostatic hypotension (a drop in blood pressure that can cause dizziness or fainting) during exercise performed while upright, so cycling or swimming may be better choices than walking or running. Beware of exercising in very hot or cold climates, and drink plenty of water.

RETINOPATHY

Some types of physical activity increase the risk of a hemorrhage in the eye or a detached retina. Avoid activities that involve a lot of jarring or straining, such as jogging or weight lifting.

PERIPHERAL NEUROPATHY

If you can't feel your feet, how will you know if you're pounding the pavement too hard? People with serious loss of sensation in the lower limbs should not overdo weight-bearing exercise. Repetitive, intense pressure on the feet can cause ulcers. You may also fail to realize that you have broken a foot bone. If you have nerve damage that limits feeling in your feet, low-impact exercise, such as swimming, cycling, or rowing, may be the best choice.

CARDIO EXERCISES

MARCH IN PLACE

Marching in place is a low-intensity, moderate-impact exercise. Like other cardio activities, it increases the heart rate to strengthen the heart and lungs while also increasing circulation throughout the body. If neuropathy of the feet is present, do seated.

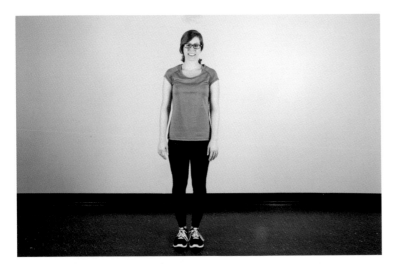

STEP 1

Stand (or sit) tall with abdominals pulled in.

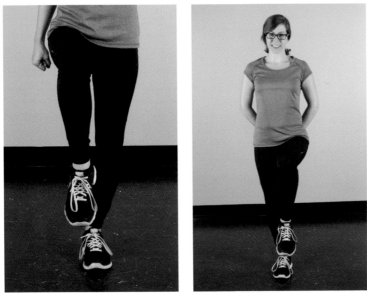

STEP 2

March in place for 1–2 minutes.

STEP 3

For added intensity,
swing arms.

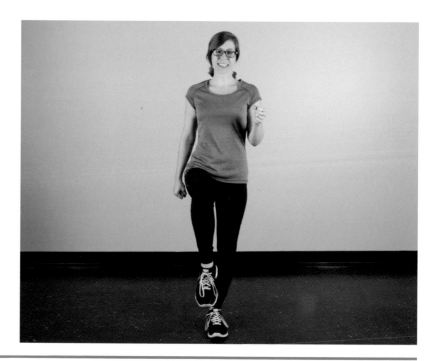

RUN IN PLACE

Running in place is a moderate-intensity, moderate-impact exercise. Avoid this exercise if neuropathy of the feet is present.

STEP 1

Stand tall with
abdominals pulled in.

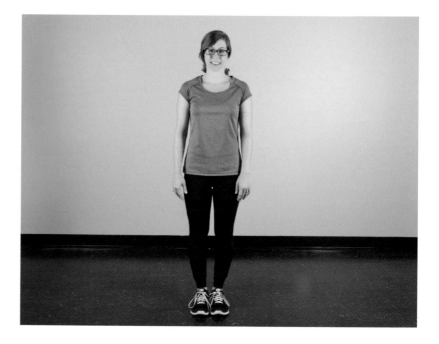

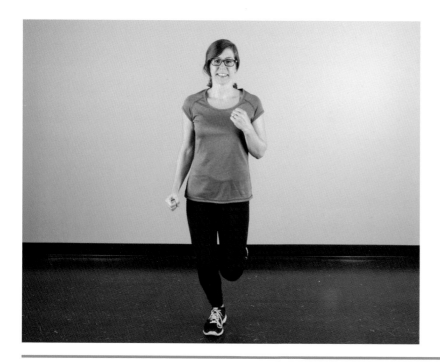

STEP 2

Run in place for
1–2 minutes.

STEP 3

For added intensity,
swing arms.

HEEL TAPS

Heel taps are a low-intensity, low-impact exercise. Along with providing cardiovascular benefits, heel taps also aid in stretching the back of legs and ankles.

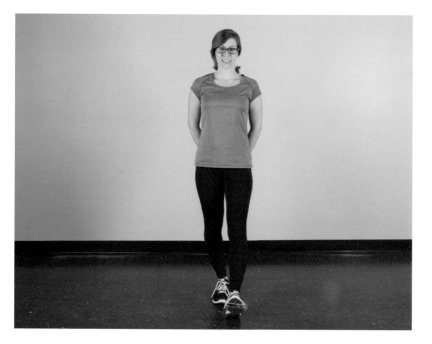

STEP 1

Stand (or sit) tall with
abdominals pulled in.

Using a quick pace,
alternating legs,
tap heels on floor
for 1–2 minutes.

STEP 2

As you do this exercise, keep toe pointed to ceiling.

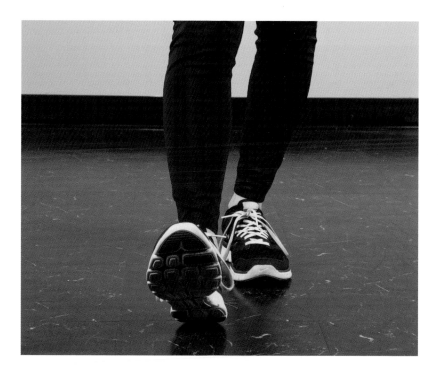

STEP 3

For added intensity, add an arm reach to ceiling.

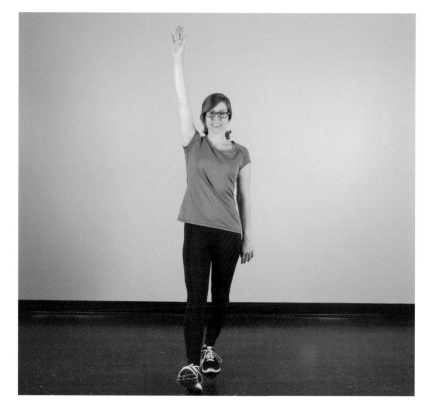

TOE TAPS

Toe taps are a low-intensity, low-impact exercise. Along with providing cardiovascular benefits, toe taps also aid in stretching the front of legs and ankles.

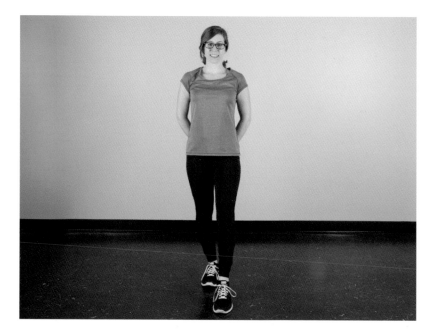

STEP 1

Stand (or sit) tall with abdominals pulled in.

Using a quick pace and alternating legs, tap toes on floor for 1–2 minutes.

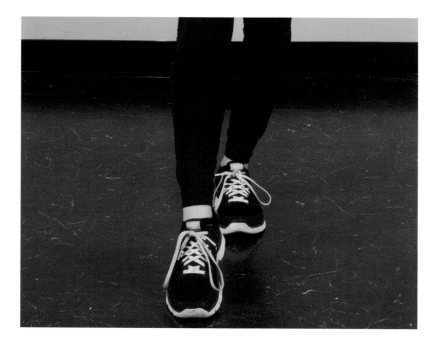

STEP 2

As you do this exercise, keep toe pointed to floor.

STEP 3

For added intensity,
add an arm reach
to ceiling.

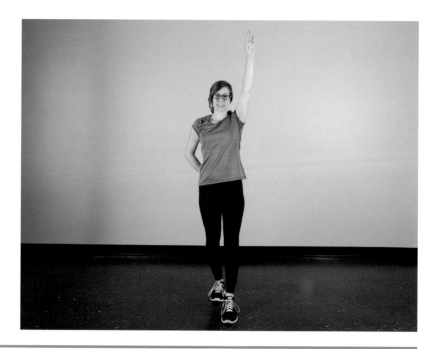

JUMP ROPE

Jumping rope is a moderate-intensity, high-impact exercise. This can be done with a rope or by twirling the arms without a rope. If neuropathy of the feet is present, do this exercise in a chair, omitting the rope.

STEP 1

Stand (or sit) tall with
abdominals pulled in.
Begin to hop in place,
twirling arms forward
or using a jump rope.
Hop for 1–2 minutes.

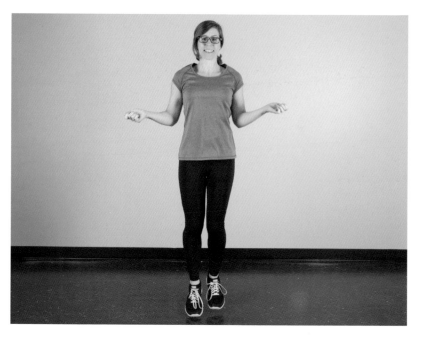

HIGH KNEES

High knees are a moderate-intensity, moderate-impact exercise. Along with providing cardiovascular benefits, high knees also aids in strengthening the hip and core muscles. If neuropathy of the feet is present, do seated.

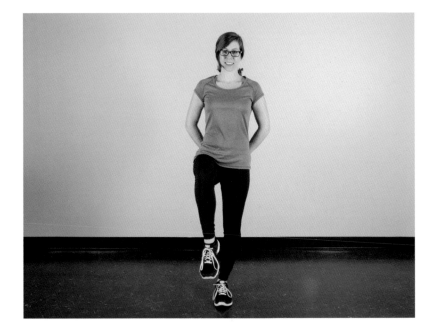

STEP 1

Stand (or sit) tall with abdominals pulled in. Alternating legs, pull knees to hip level.

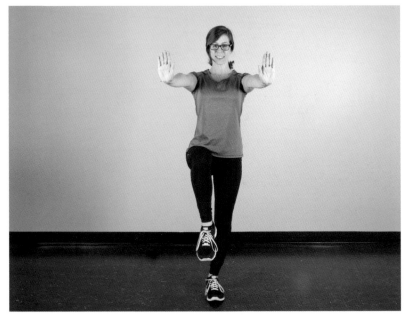

STEP 2

As you do this exercise, keep spine straight. Lift knees for 1–2 minutes.

STEP 3

For added intensity, add a forward press with arms.

SIDE STEPS

Side steps are a low-intensity, moderate-impact exercise. Along with providing cardiovascular benefits, side steps strengthen the outer and inner thighs. If neuropathy of the feet is present, do seated.

STEP 1

Stand (or sit) tall with abdominals pulled in. Step both feet to the left and then step both feet to the right.

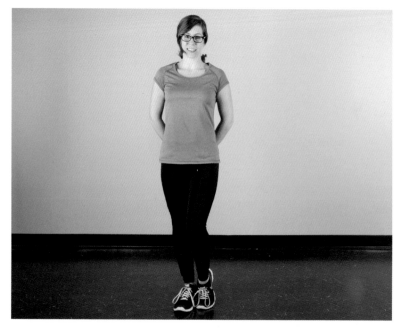

STEP 2

Step side to side for 1–2 minutes.

For added intensity, add a pulling movement with arms.

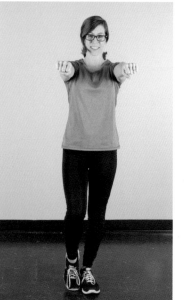 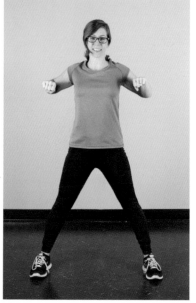

FORWARD AND BACK STEP

Stepping forward and back is a low-intensity, moderate-impact exercise. Along with providing cardiovascular benefits, stepping forward and back aids in training the walking and balance muscles of the upper leg. If neuropathy of the feet is present, do seated.

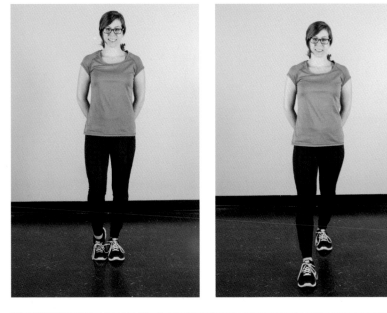

STEP 1

Stand (or sit) tall with abdominals pulled in. Step both feet forward.

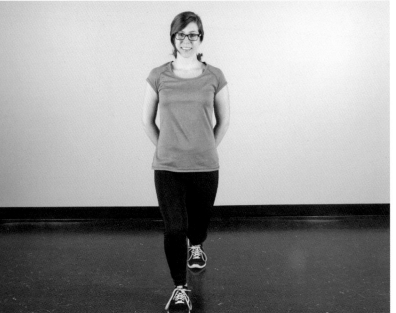

STEP 2

Step both feet back. Step forward and back for 1–2 minutes.

STEP 3

For added intensity, add a knee bend with the forward step.

JUMPING JACKS

Jumping jacks are a high-intensity, high-impact exercise. If neuropathy of the feet is present, modify exercise or do seated.

STEP 1

Stand (or sit) tall, abdominals pulled in. Jump feet out to either side while bringing arms up overhead. Then return to start. Jump for 1–2 minutes.

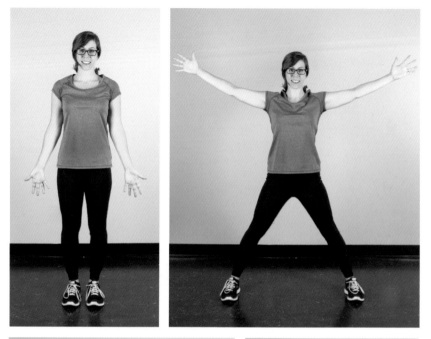

STEP 2

To modify, alternate side taps with feet while bringing arms up over head.

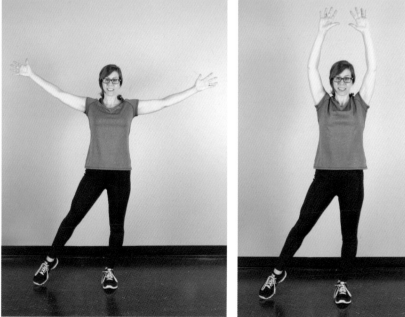

STRENGTH EXERCISES

BICEP CURLS

Bicep curls are a low-intensity, no-impact exercise. This exercise strengthens the front of the arm, the muscle used for lifting and rotating the arm outward.

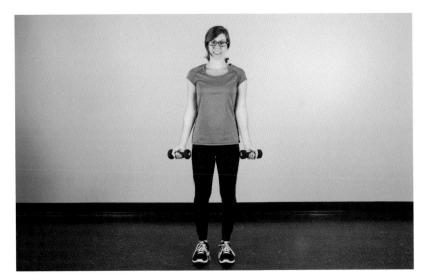

STEP 1

Stand (or sit) tall, feet at hip distance.

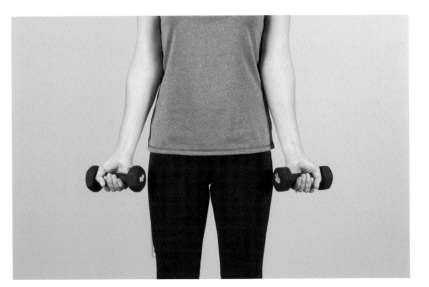

STEP 2

Put arms straight down by sides, palms facing up.

STEP 3

Keeping the elbows close to ribs, curl hands up towards shoulder.

STEP 4

The exercise can be done with one or both arms. Do 10–15 repetitions.

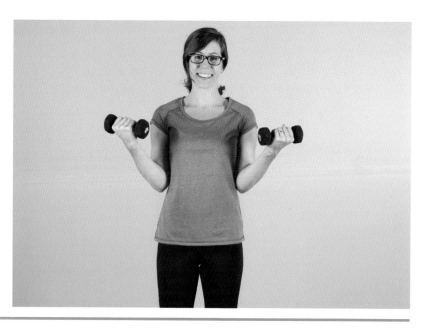

LATERAL RAISE

Lateral raises are a low-intensity, no-impact exercise. This exercise strengthens the shoulder muscles that are used for lifting and rotating the arms.

STEP 1

Stand (or sit) tall, feet at hip distance. Put arms straight down by sides, palms turned in toward body.

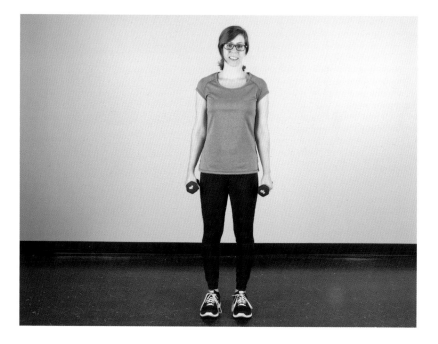

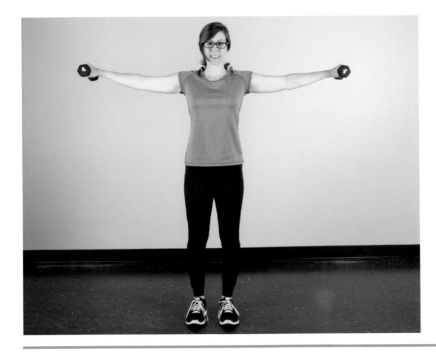

STEP 2

Lift one or both arms out to side, elbows slightly bent. Do not lift higher than the shoulder joint. Do 10–15 repetitions.

CHEST PRESS

This exercise is a low-intensity, no-impact exercise. The chest press will strengthen the chest muscles, which are important for pushing movements. This group of muscles also aids in maintaining good posture.

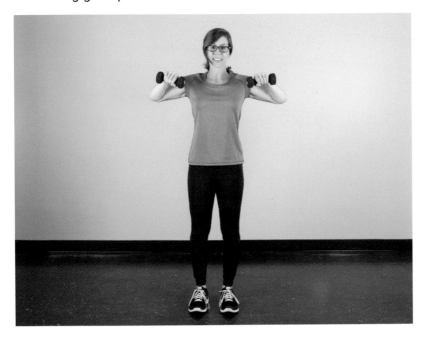

STEP 1

Stand (or sit) tall, feet at hip distance. Hands should be at chest height, palms facing down, elbows out.

STEP 2

Press arms forward.
Do not lock elbows.

STEP 3

Return to start
position. Do 10–15
repetitions.

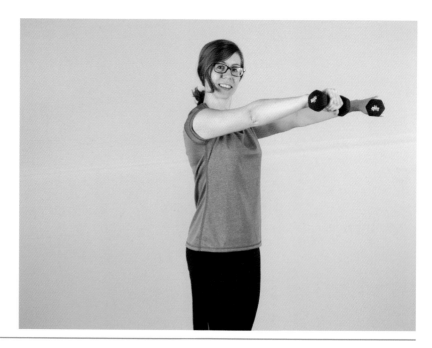

PRESS BACK

The press back exercise is a low-intensity, no-impact exercise. This exercise strengthens the upper back muscles, which are important for pulling movements. This group of muscles also aids in maintaining good posture.

STEP 1

Stand (or sit) tall, feet
at hip distance. Arms
should be straight
down by sides.

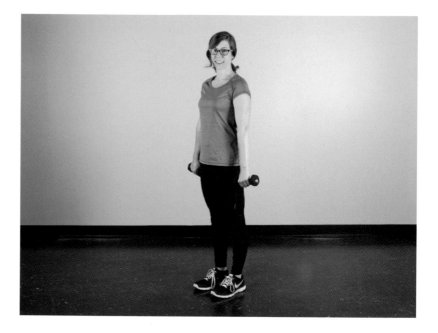

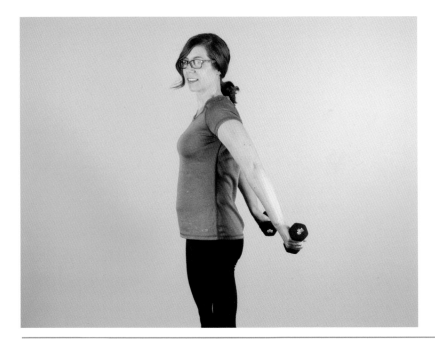

STEP 2

Face palms backward. Lift one or both arms back, squeezing shoulder blades. Keep shoulders relaxed. Do 10–15 repetitions.

SIDE LEANS

This exercise is a low-intensity, no-impact exercise. Side leans strengthen the muscles at the sides of the waist, which are part of the "core" muscle group. The core muscles aid in bending and twisting the midsection of the body. This group of muscles also contributes to posture maintenance and improving balance.

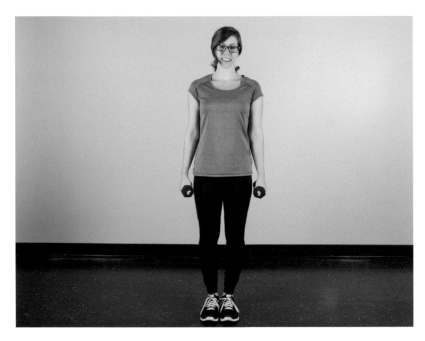

STEP 1

Stand (or sit) tall, abdominals pulled in. Arms should be straight down by sides, with the spine as straight as possible.

STEP 2

Keeping the spine long, lean to the right, crunching side of waist.

STEP 3

Do 10–15 repetitions. Repeat on other side.

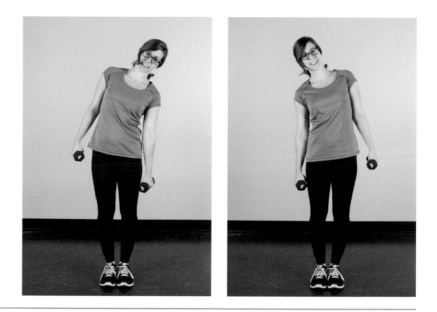

CRUNCHES

Crunches are a low-intensity, no-impact exercise. This exercise strengthens the front of the abdominals, which are part of the "core" muscle group. The front of the abdominals are the muscles responsible for bending forward; they also aid in posture maintenance and improving balance. Be cautious of this exercise if osteoporosis of the spine is present. This exercise can be done seated or laying on the floor.

IN CHAIR

STEP 1

Sit tall with abdominals pulled in.

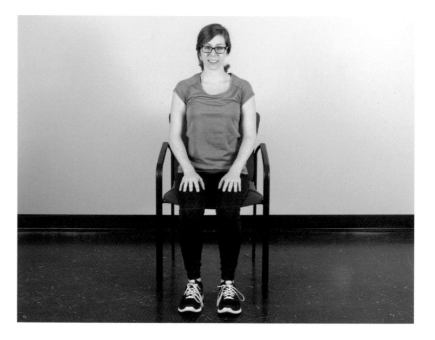

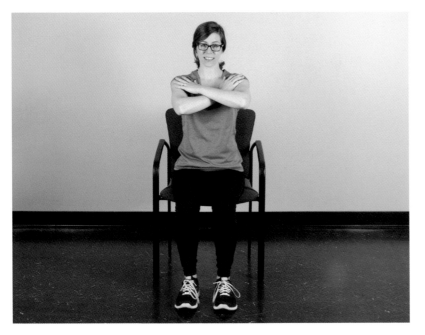

STEP 2

Cross arms in front of chest.

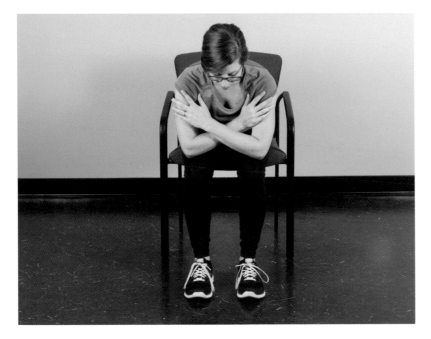

STEP 3

Keeping abdominals tight, bend forward to tap elbows to knees. Keep lower back pressing into chair. Do 10–15 repetitions.

ON THE FLOOR

STEP 1

Lie on floor, knees
bent, feet flat. Place
hands behind head for
neck support.

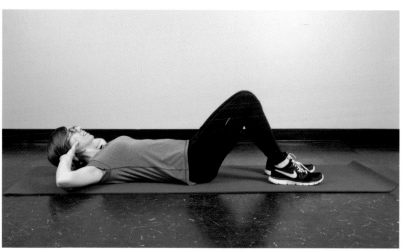

STEP 2

Keeping abdominals
tight, press lower back
into floor, curling head
and shoulders up.

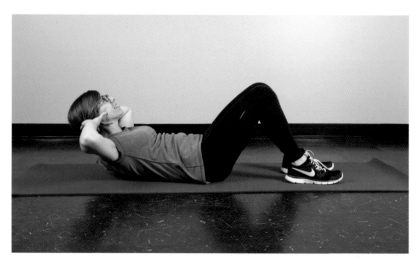

STEP 3

Do not pull on neck.
Do not lift your lower
back off floor.

STEP 4

Return to start
position. Do 10–15
repetitions.

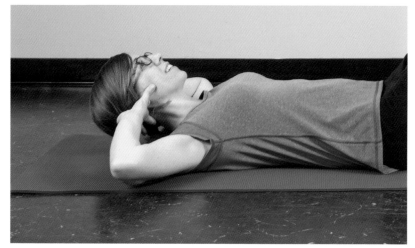

DEAD LIFT

This is a moderate-intensity, no-impact exercise. Dead lifts strengthen the muscles that run along the spine, which are important for posture maintenance and balance. Even though these muscles are located on the back, they are still an important part of the "core" muscle group. Be cautious of this exercise if lower back pain or spinal stenosis is present.

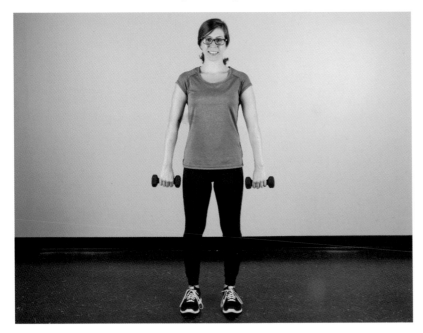

STEP 1

Stand (or sit) tall, abdominals pulled in. Arms should be hanging straight down by sides, palms facing backward.

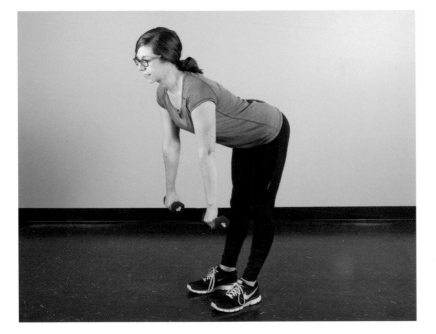

STEP 2

Keeping arms straight, bend forward with straight spine until body is at a 90 degree angle.

STEP 3

Press weight down through heels (hips, if seated). Slowly lift upper body back to start position. Do 10–15 repetitions.

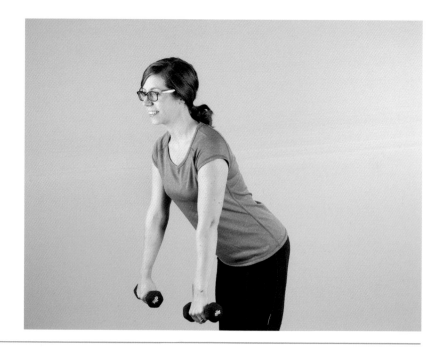

KNEE LIFT

Knee lifts are a low-intensity, low-impact exercise. This exercise strengthens the hip muscles. Be cautious of this exercise if hip pain or injury is present. An ankle weight can be used.

STEP 1

Stand (or sit) tall. Lift bent left knee to hip height.

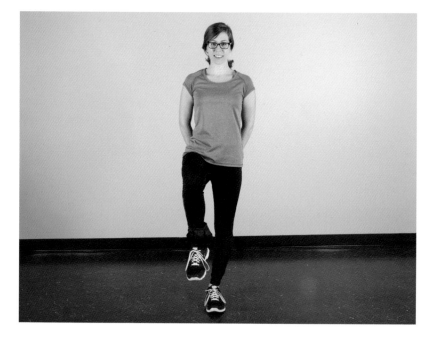

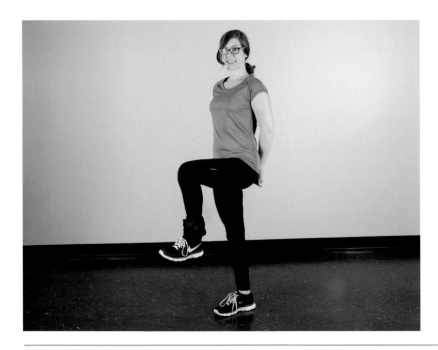

STEP 2

Keep foot flexed. Do
10–15 repetitions.

STEP 3

Repeat with
other leg.

FORWARD KICK

This exercise is a low-intensity, low-impact exercise. Forward kicks strengthen the thigh muscle.
Be cautious of this exercise if knee pain or injury is present. An ankle weight can be used.

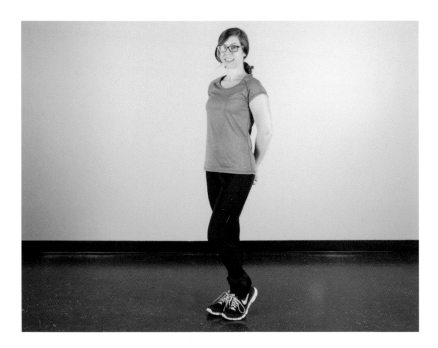

STEP 1

Stand (or sit) tall.
Slightly bend knee,
placing toe of left
foot on floor. If seated,
begin with knees bent,
feet flat.

STEP 2

Straighten leg; focus on squeezing thigh. Do 10–15 repetitions.

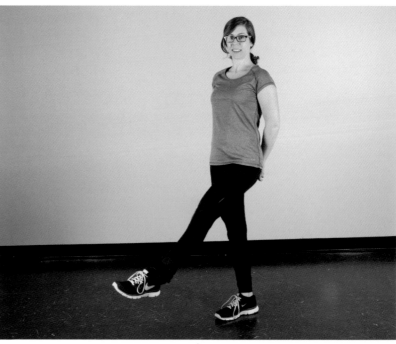

STEP 3

Repeat with other leg.

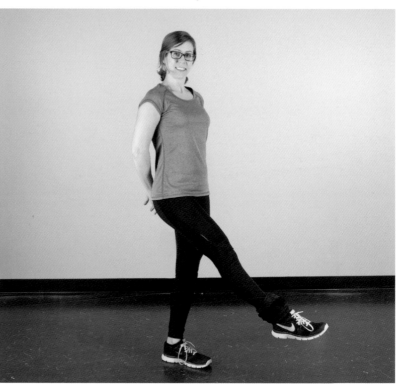

LEG CURL

The leg curl exercise is a low-intensity, no-impact exercise. This exercise strengthens the muscles at the back of the thigh, which are important for bending the knee and walking. Be cautious if knee pain or injury is present. An ankle weight can be used.

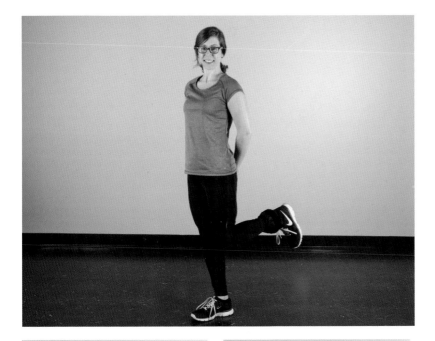

STEP 1

Stand tall, feet at hip distance. With left foot flexed, bend left knee, bringing foot backward.

STEP 2

Keep knees close together. Lower to start position. Do 10–15 repetitions. Repeat with other leg.

SIDE LEG RAISE

This exercise is a low-intensity, no-impact exercise. Side raises strengthen the inner and outer thigh muscles, which are important for side to side movements. Be caution of this exercise if hip pain or injury is present.

STEP 1

Stand tall, feet at hip distance. Keeping upper body tall, lift straight leg to the side. Keep foot relaxed.

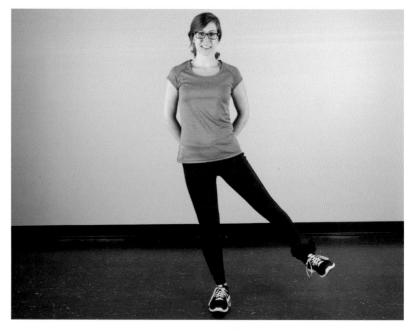

STEP 2

Return to start position. Do 10–15 repetitions.

STEP 3

Repeat with other leg.

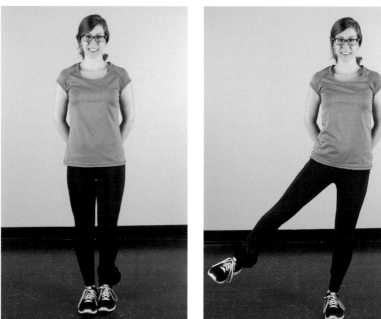

HEEL RAISES

Heel raises are a low-intensity, low-impact exercise. This exercise strengthens the calf muscles. If neuropathy of the foot is present, do this exercise seated.

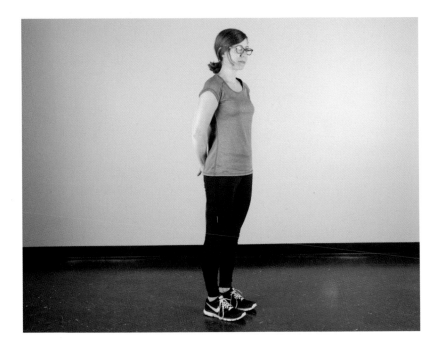

STEP 1

Stand (or sit) tall, feet at hip distance.

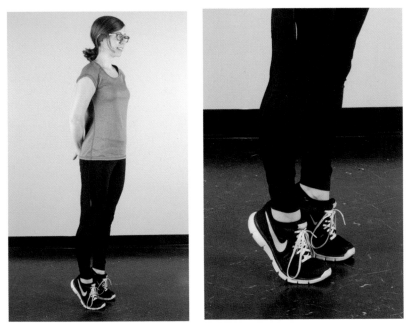

STEP 2

Keeping upper body tall and legs straight (knees bent, if seated), lift one or both heels off the ground. Do 10–15 repetitions.

SQUATS

Squats are a moderate-intensity, no-impact exercise. Squats challenge all of the muscles of the upper leg, which are important for the fundamental movements of the lower body, such as walking, bending the knees, lifting the legs, and getting in and out of a chair. If hip or knee problems are present, do partial squats or avoid this exercise.

STEP 1

Stand with feet at hip distance. Pull in abdominals to protect lower back.

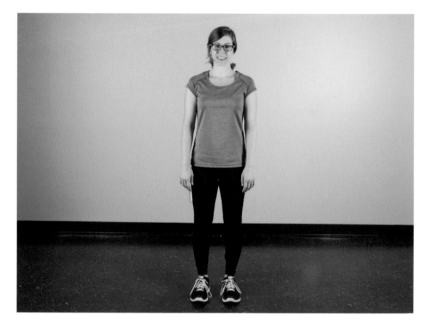

STEP 2

Bend knees and move hips back, as if sitting in a chair. Do not take knees further forward than toes.

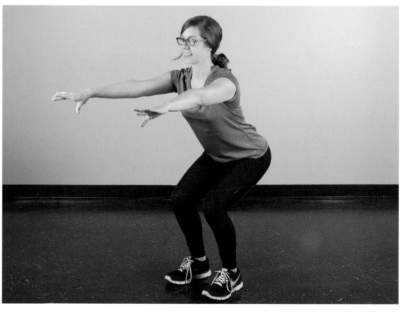

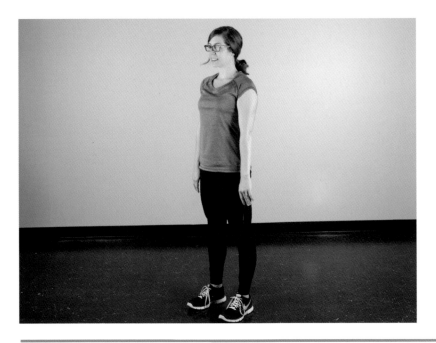

STEP 3

Press weight through heels to return to standing position. Do 10–15 repetitions.

LUNGES

Lunges are a moderate-intensity, no-impact exercise. This exercise strengthens the muscles of the thigh. If knee pain or injury is present, avoid this exercise.

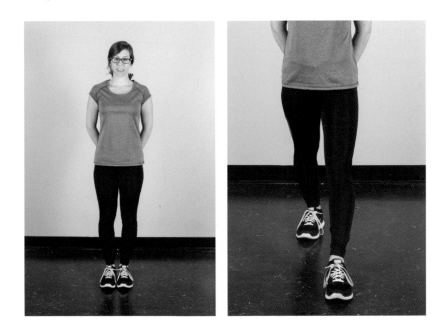

STEP 1

Stand tall with feet at hip distance. Step left foot forward into staggered stance.

STEP 2

Keeping upper body tall, bend both knees to 90 degrees. Do not let knees go past the toes.

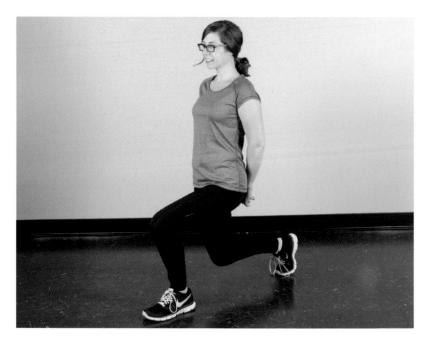

STEP 3

Return to standing position. Do 10–15 repetitions.

STEP 4

Repeat with other leg.

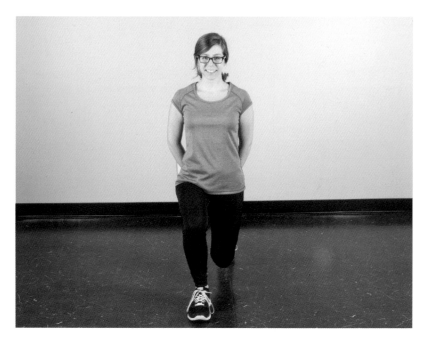

FITNESS BALL

PELVIC CIRCLES

This exercise is designed to enhance core strength and improve balance. Pelvic circles are low intensity and add no impact to the spine. This exercise is a challenge for those with balance issues, so use the ball with caution.

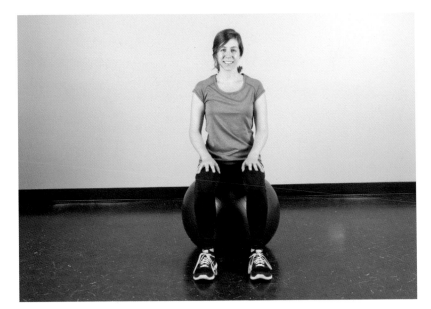

STEP 1

Sit on a stability ball with feet flat on the floor, spine tall. Pull the abdominals in toward the spine.

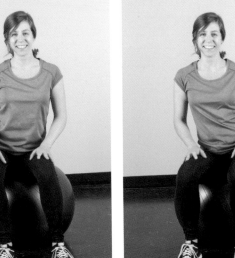

STEP 2

Make a circular motion with the hips moving in a clockwise direction. Do 15 repetitions, then repeat going the other direction.

HIP EXTENSIONS

Hip extensions target the hips and legs, both important muscles for walking. Adding the stability ball engages the core muscles and adds a balance challenge to the exercise. This is a no-impact, moderate-intensity exercise.

STEP 1

Lie flat on your back with ankles resting on a stability ball, legs straight.

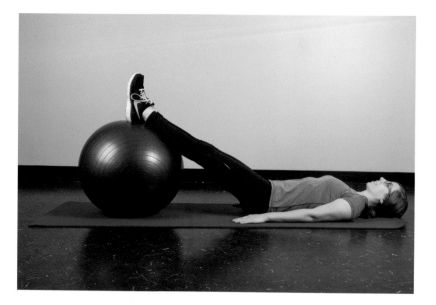

STEP 2

Keeping legs straight and abdominals contracted, lift hips towards ceiling. Keep neck and shoulders relaxed.

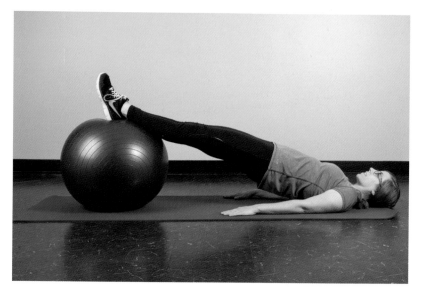

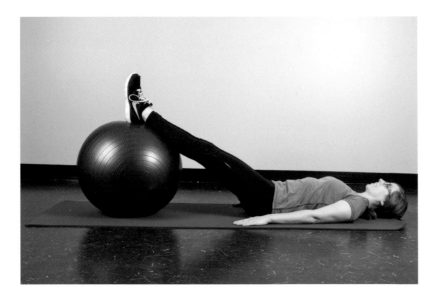

STEP 3

Pause for 1 count at the top of the lift. With firm abdominals, lower the hips back to the floor. Do 10–15 repetitions.

BACK EXTENSIONS

This exercise is a low-intensity back exercise that helps to improve posture and core strength. Back extensions are of moderate impact to the spine, so people with spinal stenosis should avoid this exercise.

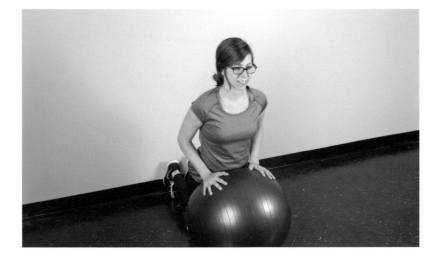

STEP 1

Bring the ball to an area with a wall nearby. Kneel in front of the ball. Lean forward, placing abdominals on the ball.

STEP 2

Straighten legs, securing feet against a wall.

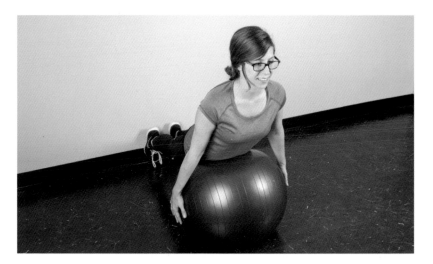

STEP 3

Round the upper body forward so it is draped over the ball.

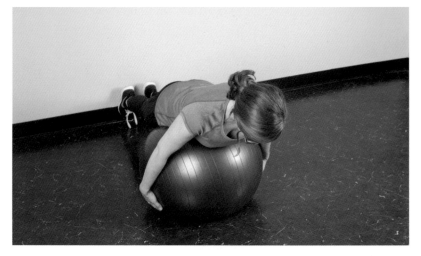

STEP 4

Lift the head and shoulders up until upper body is in line with lower body. Do not extend beyond a straight spine. Do 10–15 repetitions.

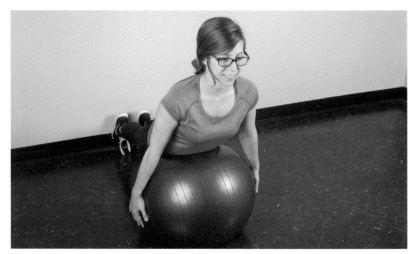

WALL SQUAT

Wall squats are a moderate-intensity, moderate-impact exercise designed to strengthen the legs. This exercise also engages the core muscles. If knee pain is present, only squat halfway or to tolerance. Use caution if suffering from peripheral neuropathy.

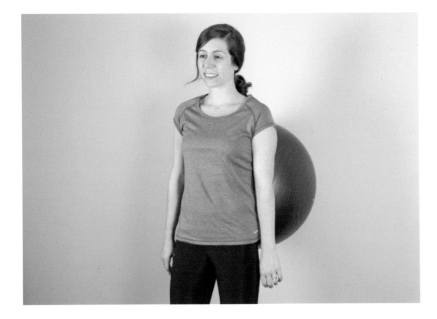

STEP 1

Stand with back to wall, ball resting against lower back. Feet should be hip distance apart.

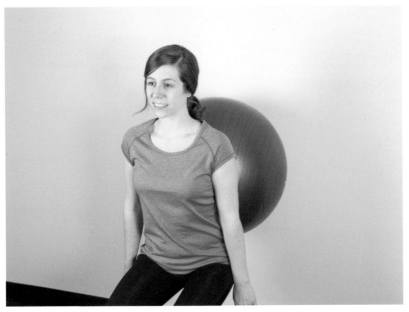

STEP 2

Keeping upper body straight and abdominals contracted, lower the hips and bend the knees. Be sure that knees are not going past toes.

STEP 3

Press weight down through the heels to press back up to standing.

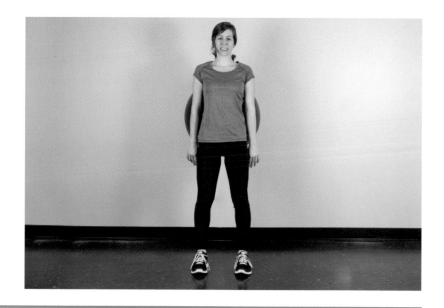

BRIDGE

This is a low-intensity, no-impact exercise targeting the lower body. The addition of the ball engages the core muscles and aids in balance training. Use caution if suffering from peripheral neuropathy.

STEP 1

Sit on ball with feet flat on floor.

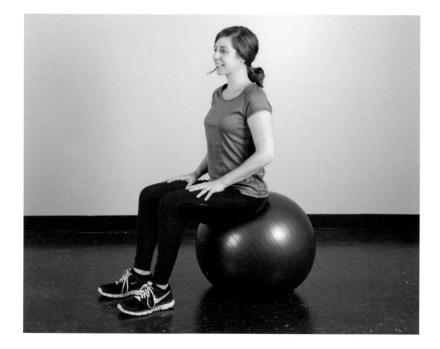

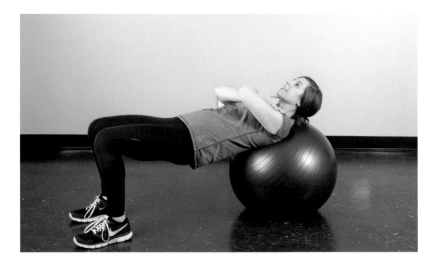

STEP 2

Walk the feet forward until upper body is resting on the ball, with knees bent at 90 degrees. Cross hands over chest.

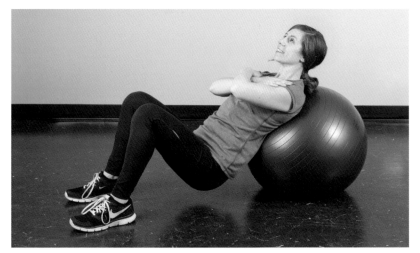

STEP 3

With tight abdominals, lower the hips until just above the floor.

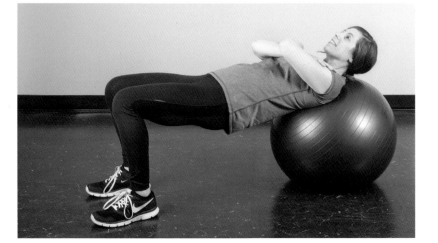

STEP 4

Keeping abdominals firm, press through the heels to lift the hips back to start position. Do 15 repetitions.

LIFT AND SQUEEZE

The lift and squeeze is a moderate-intensity, no-impact exercise. This exercise targets the inner thigh muscles that aid in maintaining knee and hip alignment. The core muscles are also challenged while doing this exercise. This exercise is safe for all fitness levels.

STEP 1

Lie flat on back with feet on either side of stability ball.

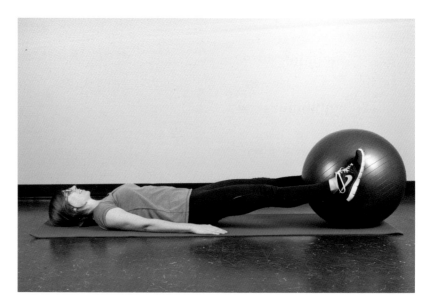

STEP 2

Squeeze the feet against ball and lift off the ground. Keep lower back pressing into floor or mat, abdominals pulled in.

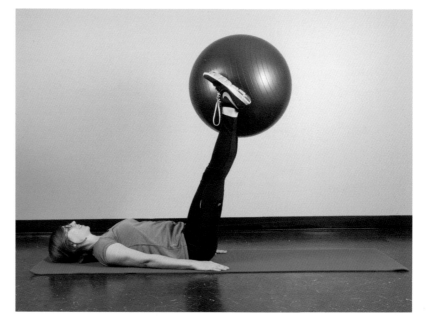

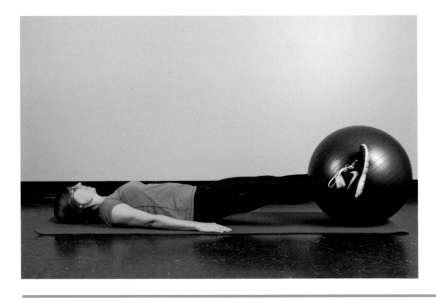

STEP 3

Keeping the feet squeezed against ball, slowly lower back to ground. Do 10–15 repetitions.

AB ROLL

This is a moderate-intensity activity targeting the abdominal muscles. Ab rolls can put some strain on the back and knees, so avoid this exercise if any pain occurs.

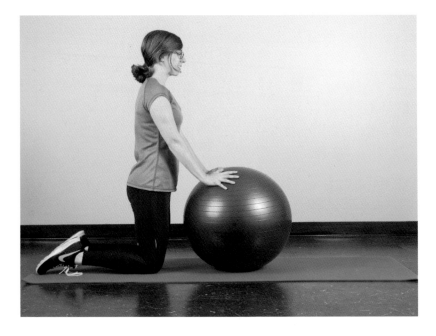

STEP 1

Kneel on floor in front of ball with hands resting on the ball. Keep your elbows bent and hands parallel.

STEP 2

Tightening abdominals, roll ball as far forward as comfortable, keeping knees on floor. Keep spine straight. Do not let hips drop.

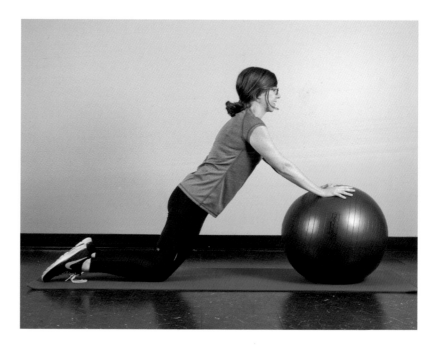

STEP 3

Pause in rolled out position for one deep breath. Slowly roll back to start. Do 10–15 repetitions.

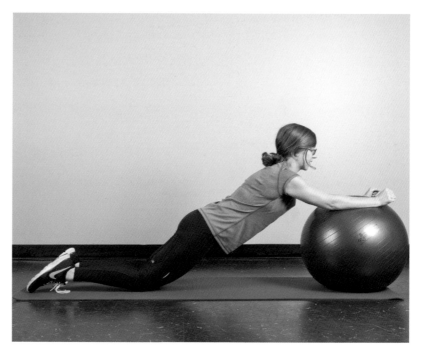

LEG EXTENSIONS

Leg extensions on a stability ball are a double duty strength and balance exercise; they target the thigh muscles and the core. This low-intensity, no-impact exercise is safe for all fitness levels.

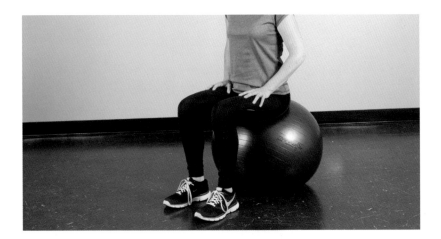

STEP 1

Sit on ball with feet flat on floor. Place hands on thighs. For more stability, place hands on either side of ball.

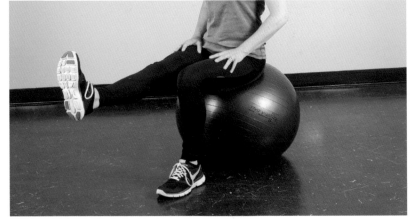

STEP 2

Sitting tall, lift right leg straight out, toes pointing to ceiling.

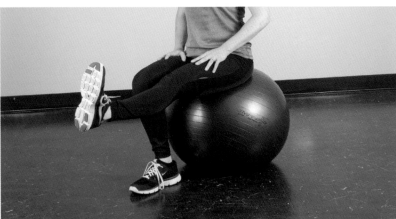

STEP 3

Lower to start position. Do 10–15 repetitions. Repeat with other leg.

STEP 4

Lift arms to create a greater balance challenge.

KNEE LIFTS

Knee lifts on a stability ball target the hip muscles as well as the core and back. This exercise is low intensity and is a double duty exercise that helps not only strength but also balance and posture. This exercise is safe for all fitness levels.

STEP 1

Sit on ball with feet flat on floor. Place hands on thighs.

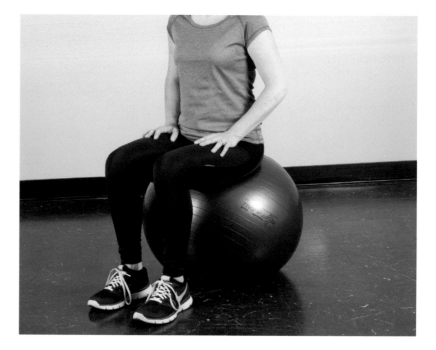

STEP 2

Sit tall with abdominals tight. Lift knee as high as possible. Do not round forward, but keep a long spine.

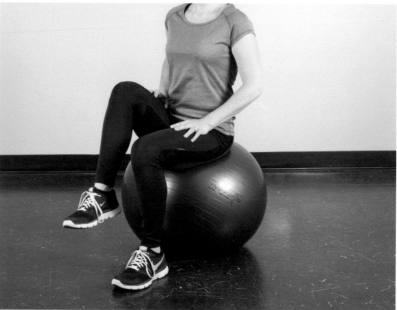

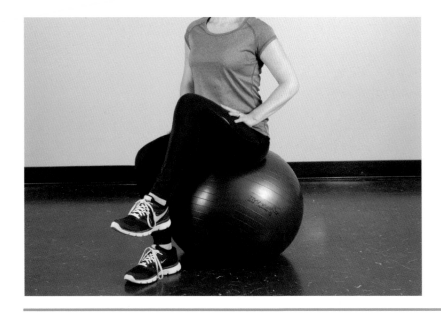

STEP 3

Lower to start position. Do 10–15 repetitions. Repeat with other leg.

STEP 4

Lift arms to create a greater balance challenge.

CALF RAISES

Strong calves are an important element for good balance and proper knee and ankle alignment. Calf raises on the stability ball are a low-intensity, low-impact way to strengthen the calf muscles while also working the core muscles and improving posture. This exercise may not be suitable for people with peripheral neuropathy in the feet.

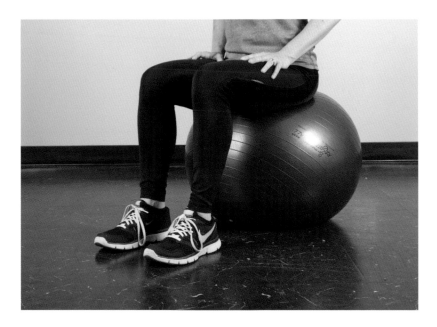

STEP 1

Sit on the ball with feet at hip distance (feet together for increased balance challenge). Keep spine long and ab-dominals pulled in.

STEP 2

Lift left heel off ground, pause. Lower to start position. Do 10–15 repetitions. Repeat with other leg.

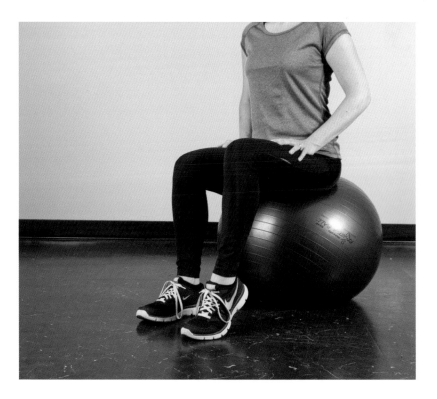

STEP 3

For added challenge, do both legs.

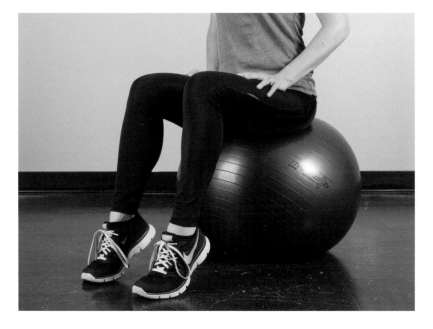

BICEP CURLS

This is a low-intensity, no-impact exercise. Bicep curls target the muscle on the front of the arm. This muscle is important for lifting and pulling. The addition of the ball helps with core strength and balance. If hand strength is compromised because of neuropathy of the hand, use caution. This exercise can also be done with wrist weights. Do one arm at a time to decrease the challenge, if needed.

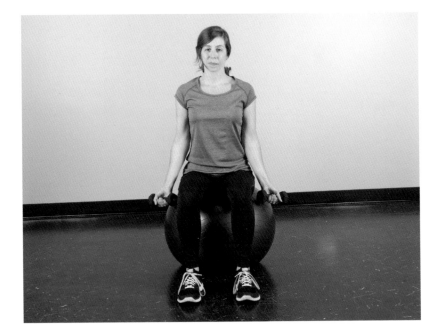

STEP 1

Sit on ball with feet at hip distance (feet closer together for added balance challenge). Keep spine long and abdominals pulled in. Hold a 5–10 lb weight in each hand, palms facing up.

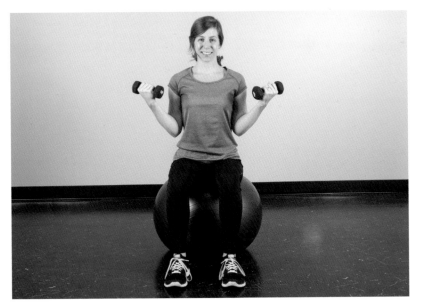

STEP 2

Keeping elbows close to body, curl hands up toward shoulders, with palms facing up to ceiling. Do 10–15 repetitions.

CHEST FLY

Chest fly exercises strengthen the muscles in the front of the chest. These muscles are key for good posture. This exercise is a moderate-intensity, no-impact exercise and is safe for all fitness levels. The addition of the ball incorporates core strength and balance.

STEP 1

Sit on ball, feet at hip distance. Hold a 5–10 lb weight in each hand. Walk feet forward until upper back is resting on ball.

STEP 2

Straighten arms over head so hands are directly over the face, palms in. Arms should be nearly straight, keeping slight bend in elbows.

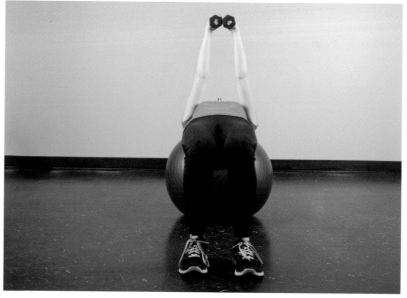

STEP 3

Lower arms out to sides, keeping elbows slightly bent.

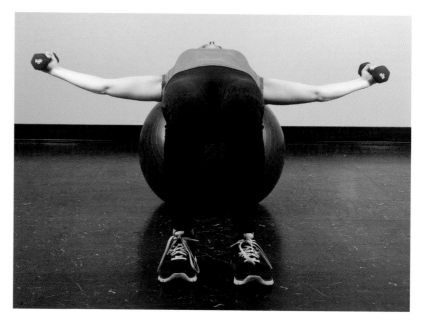

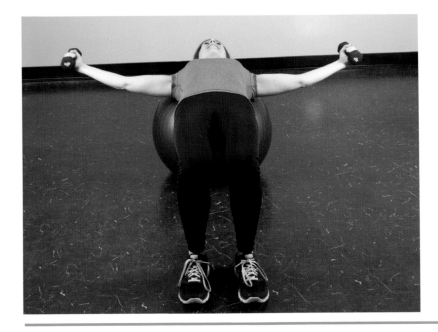

STEP 4

Return to start position. Do 10–15 repetitions.

TRICEP EXTENSION

This is a low-intensity, no-impact exercise. Tricep extensions work the back of the arms, strengthening the muscles in charge of pulling and pressing. The addition of the ball incorporates core strength and balance.

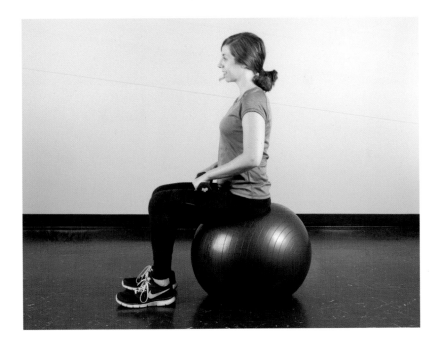

STEP 1

Sit on ball, feet at hip distance. Hold a 5–10 lb weight in each hand.

STEP 2

Walk feet forward until upper back is resting on ball. Keep hips lifted.

STEP 3

Straighten arms overhead so hands are directly over the face, palms in. Arms should be straight.

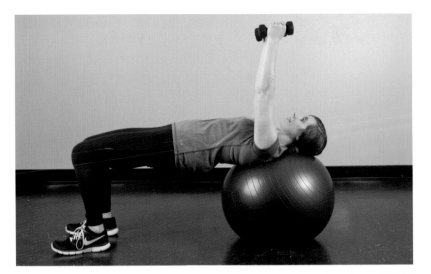

STEP 4

Bend elbows to 90 degrees, lowering hands behind head.

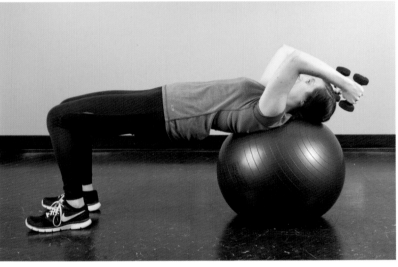

STEP 5

Press back to start position. Do 10–15 repetitions.

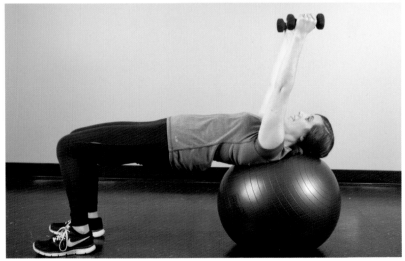

YOGA POSES

MOUNTAIN POSE

Mountain Pose is a low-intensity pose that is safe for all fitness levels. This exercise is beneficial for improving posture and lower body strength, as well as strengthening the core.

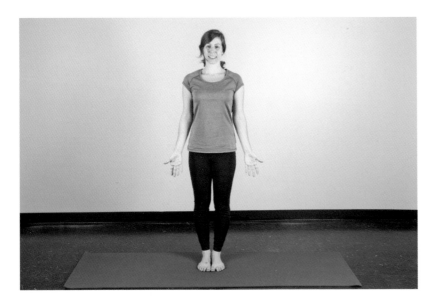

STEP 1

Stand tall with feet at hip distance. Tuck tailbone in and pull abdominals in toward spine. Relax shoulders; let arms hang by sides with palms facing out.

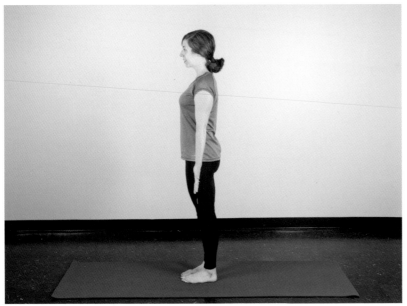

STEP 2

Reach crown of head toward the ceiling while pushing heels down into floor. Hold for 5 breaths.

LOW LUNGE/HIGH LUNGE

Low Lunge is a low-intensity balance pose. This pose may be difficult for people with peripheral neuropathy, so practice with caution. Low Lunge strengthens the lower body as well as relieving pressure caused by sciatica. High Lunge is a moderate-intensity balance pose that aids in stretching the groin and strengthens the legs.

STEP 1

Begin in Mountain Pose. Step right foot back into a wide leg stance.

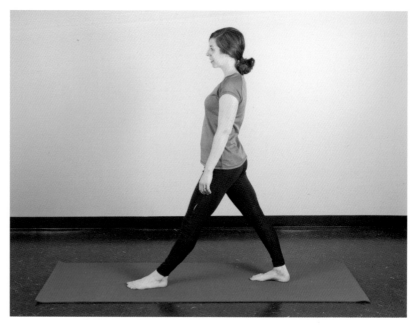

STEP 2

Bend left knee to 90 degrees while lowering left knee to floor. Straighten left leg as much as possible, pressing hips down toward floor.

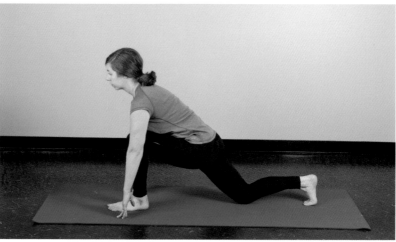

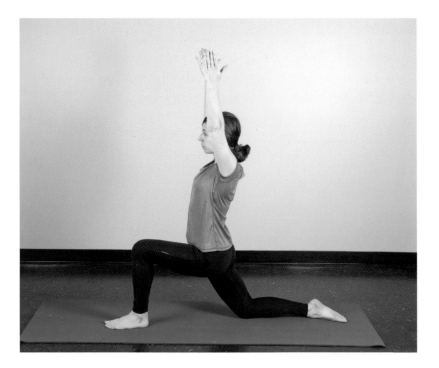

STEP 3

Place both hands on left knee and straighten upper body. Inhale while sweeping both hands up to the ceiling. For an added balance challenge, look up. Hold for 3 deep breaths. Repeat with left leg.

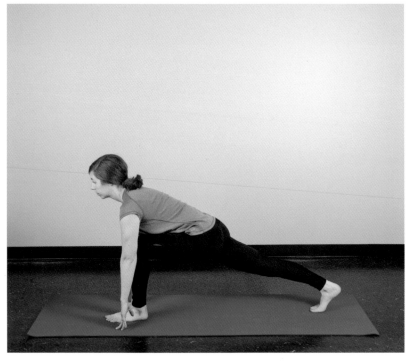

STEP 4

To move into High Lunge, place fingers on floor for stability and press right leg straight. Repeat steps 2 and 3.

DOWNWARD FACING DOG

Downward Facing Dog is a moderate-intensity pose. It strengthens and stretches muscles of the entire body and aids in preventing osteoporosis. Benefits include improved digestion and increased energy. Be cautious practicing this pose if carpal tunnel syndrome is present.

STEP 1

Begin on hands and knees with wrists under shoulders and knees under hips.

STEP 2

Curling toes under, press hips up to ceiling.

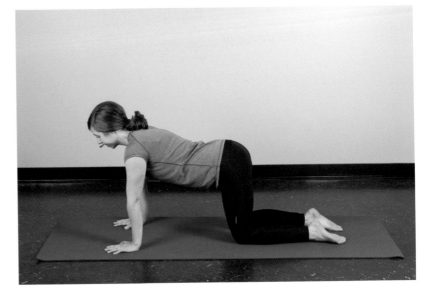

STEP 3

Adjust body so arms are straight with palms pressing firmly into floor.

STEP 4

Continue to lift hips up while pressing heels down. Bend knees slightly if pain is felt in legs. Hold for 5 breaths.

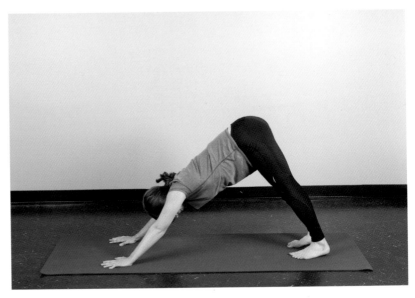

140

WARRIOR POSE

Warrior Pose is a moderate-intensity pose designed to strengthen and stretch the legs and ankles. This pose also facilitates core strengthening and balance training. If problems with the neck are present do not turn to look over the fingertips, but keep head forward.

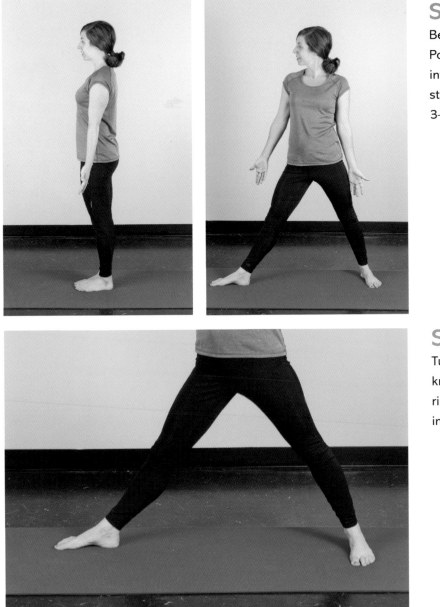

STEP 1

Begin in Mountain Pose. Step feet into wide leg stance, about 3–4 feet apart.

STEP 2

Turn left foot and knee outward, while right foot remains in place.

STEP 3

Inhale to sweep
arms out to sides
and look over
fingertips.

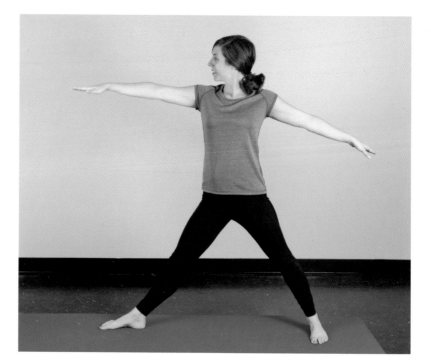

STEP 4

Bend front leg to 90
degrees. Keep upper
body very tall.

STEP 5

Keeping back leg
very straight, push
outside edge of
back foot into floor.
Hold for 3 breaths.

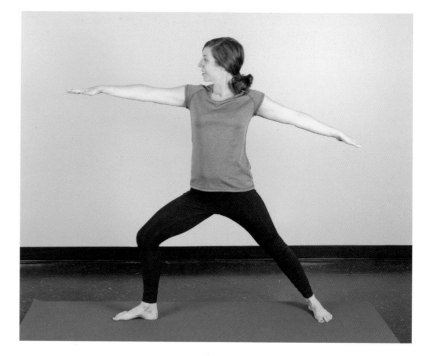

TREE POSE

This pose is a moderate-intensity balance pose. Tree Pose strengthens the ankles, calves, and thighs. It also promotes strengthening of the core and back. Tree Pose also helps improve focus.

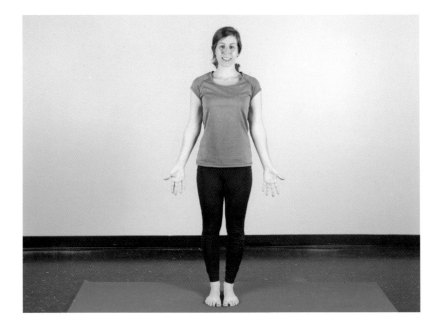

STEP 1

Begin in Mountain Pose. Rest bottom of right foot against left ankle with knee turned out. If turning knee out causes pain in hip, keep knee pointing forward.

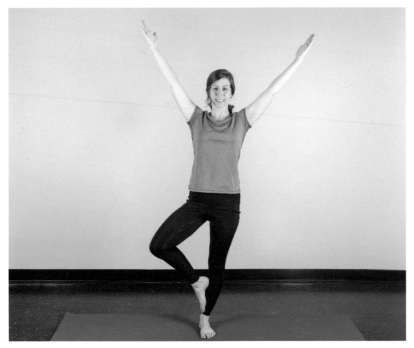

STEP 2

Keep spine long and abdominals firm. Pull right foot up to shin or thigh. Do not rest foot against knee. Reach both hands up to ceiling. Hold for 3 deep breaths. Repeat with other leg.

MOON POSE

Moon pose is a low-intensity pose used to stretch the arms and the sides of the waist.

STEP 1

Begin in Mountain Pose. Interlace fingers and turn palms down.

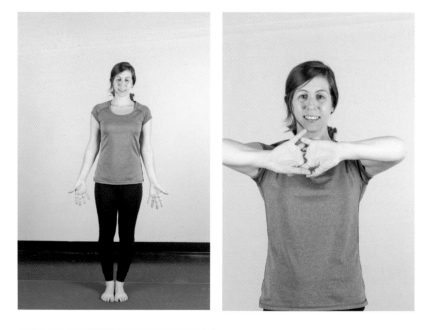

STEP 2

Inhale hands up over head, palms facing up.

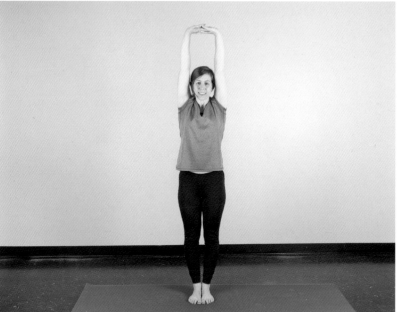

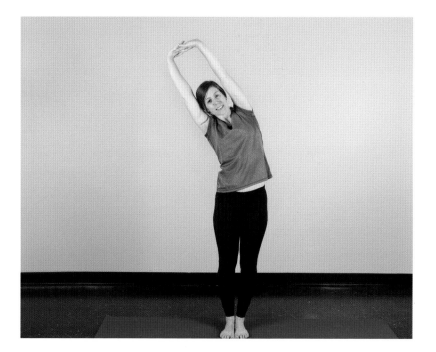

STEP 3

With hands reaching up, lean upper body to the right. Hold for 3 deep breaths.

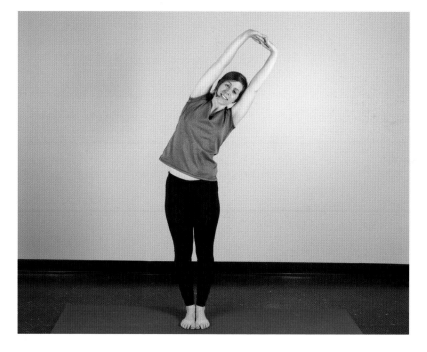

STEP 4

Repeat on left side.

CAT/COW

This flow series is low intensity and aids in strengthening and stretching the low back and core muscles. Cat and Cow is a pose used to practice pairing breath with movement, which helps relieve anxiety. Because this pose is done on hands and knees, be cautious if knee or wrist pain occurs.

ON A MAT

STEP 1

Begin on hands and knees, with wrists under shoulders and knees under hips.

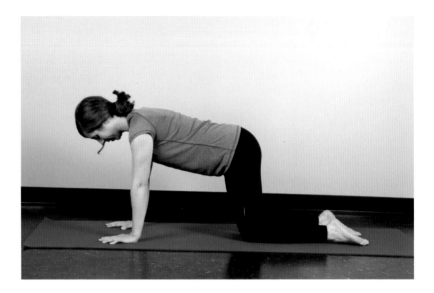

STEP 2

Inhale while rounding the back.

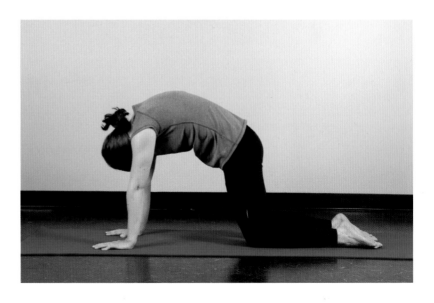

146

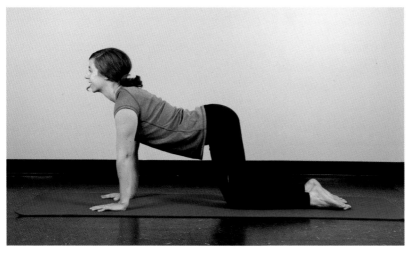

STEP 3

Exhale while pressing hands and knees into floor, arching back, and looking upward. Each breath pattern equals one set. Continue for 5 sets.

IN A CHAIR

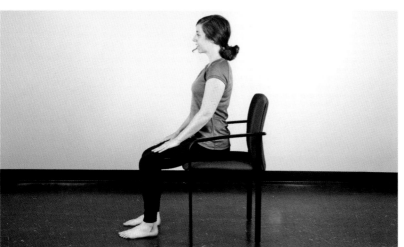

STEP 1

Begin seated in chair with hands on thighs.

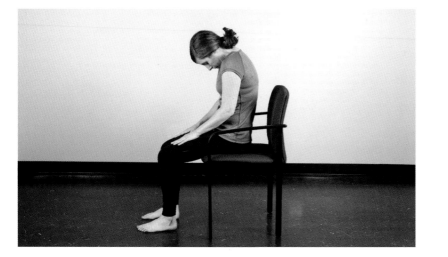

STEP 2

Inhale while rounding the back.

STEP 3

Exhale while arching back and looking up to ceiling. Each breath pattern equals one set. Continue for 5 sets.

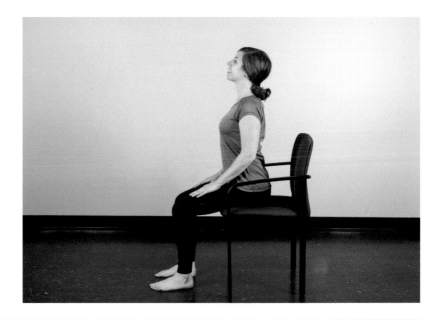

TRIANGLE POSE

Triangle Pose is a moderate-intensity pose that stretches and strengthens the lower body. It is also helpful in relieving anxiety and stress. If neck pain occurs in this stretch, do not look up at ceiling, but keep head pointing forward.

STEP 1

Begin in Mountain Pose. Step feet into wide leg stance, about 3–4 feet apart. Position feet as shown here.

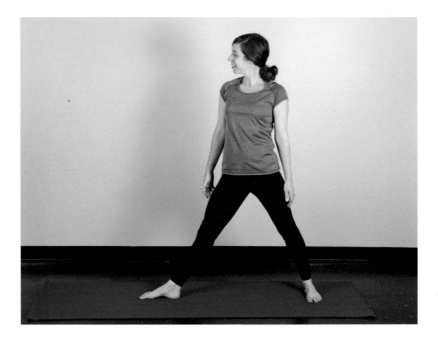

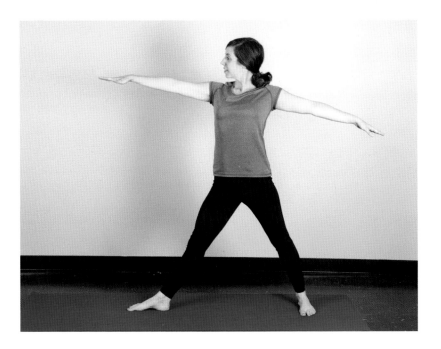

STEP 2

Inhale arms out
to sides.

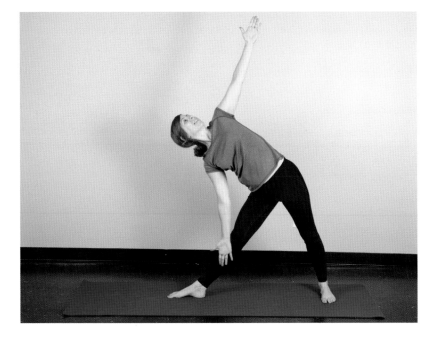

STEP 3

Exhale to reach
right hand to shin
or ankle. Left arm
reaches up to the
ceiling. If it's com-
fortable, turn the
head to look up at
left arm. Keep back
straight, tailbone
tucked under.

STEP 4

Hold for 3 deep breaths, then repeat on other side.

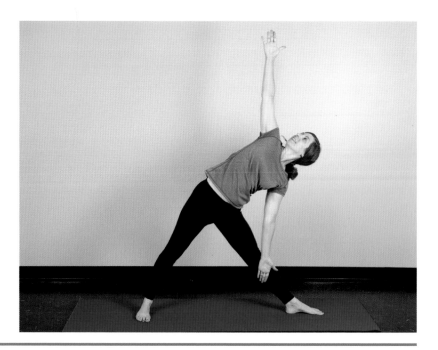

BOUND ANGEL POSE

This pose is a low-intensity pose that promotes stimulation of the heart and improves circulation. Other benefits include decreased stress, anxiety, and depression. Bound Angel Pose focuses on stretching the inner thigh, groin, and knees. If hip, groin, or knee pain is present, sit up on a pillow or yoga block.

STEP 1

Sit tall with feet flat on floor, knees bent.

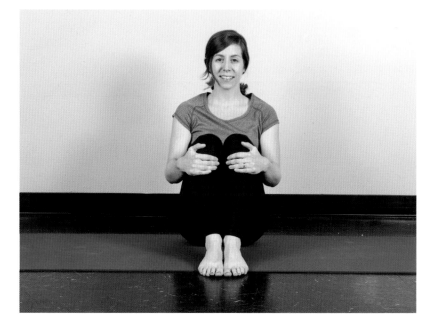

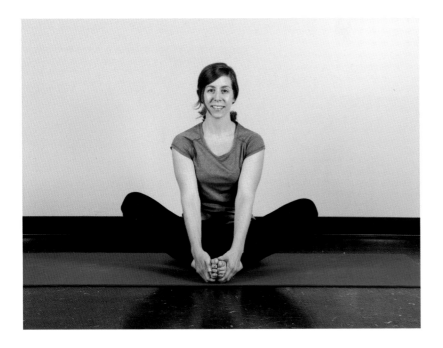

STEP 2

Open knees out to sides and pull heels in toward pelvis.

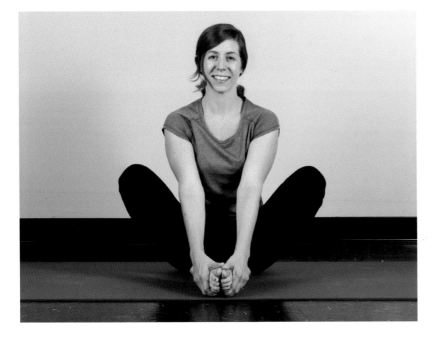

STEP 3

Place hands around feet.

STEP 4

Round forward, bringing head towards feet. Hold for 3 deep breaths.

UNDERSTANDING YOUR DRUG OPTIONS

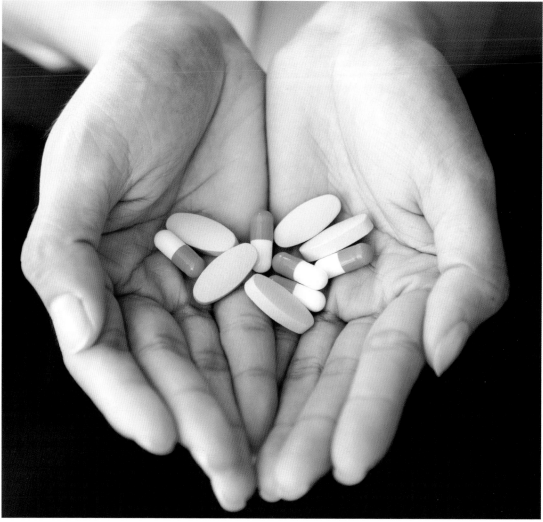

Okay, so perhaps your efforts at treating your type 2 diabetes through dietary changes, exercise, and weight loss weren't enough to get your blood sugar into a safe range. Or perhaps they did help for a few months or even years, but now your blood sugar levels have begun to creep upward again. If you don't do something more to get your disease under control, you may soon begin to feel the effects of your raging blood sugar levels from head to toe.

Fortunately, your doctor can prescribe one or more medications that—when added to your ongoing diet and exercise regimen—can help. (Drugs for treating diabetes are used *in addition to,* not in place of, lifestyle changes.)

Most of the medications that are used to treat type 2 diabetes work by doing one or more of the following:

- decreasing the amount of glucose that the liver releases into the bloodstream
- prompting the pancreas to increase the supply of insulin
- making the body's cells more sensitive to insulin
- reducing the rate at which the body absorbs sugar from food
- controlling appetite and blunting huge glucose spikes following meals

The good news: The majority of these drugs come in the form of a pill. The not-as-good news: Many of them can cause side effects ranging from bothersome to debilitating,

NO TIME TO WAIT

If you've recently been diagnosed with type 2 diabetes and your blood sugars are very high, your doctor may prescribe diabetes medication in conjunction with lifestyle therapies (dietary changes, exercise, and weight loss) right off the bat in order to get your numbers into a safer range more quickly.

although in many cases these effects fade over time or can be relieved by adjusting the dosage of the drug. You will probably have to take whatever drug or combination of drugs your doctor prescribes on an ongoing basis, perhaps even for the rest of your life. But remember: Research shows that controlling blood sugar can postpone or prevent frightening diabetes complications.

ORAL DRUGS

The following types of medication act in different ways, but all work toward moving blood sugar levels into a healthier range.

Biguanides

Includes: metformin (Fortamet, Glucophage and Glucophage XR, Glumetza, Riomet)
The single drug in this category is metformin, and it is currently the most frequently prescribed medication for treating type 2 diabetes in the world. Metformin is a multi-talented drug. For example, one way it helps control blood sugar is by making muscle cells more sensitive to insulin, so they can more easily pull glucose out of the bloodstream. But metformin's main role is to get the liver to release less glucose into the bloodstream in the first place. The liver normally stockpiles glucose (which it can make by piecing together fragments of other molecules) and releases it when blood sugar levels dip too low, such as between meals, especially overnight. After all, even when you're dozing, your body still needs glucose; if your glucose dried up, your organs would shut down.

Normally, the liver slows the release of glucose when there's a lot of insulin in the blood, because that boatload of floating insulin is a sure signal that there's already plenty of sugar in the blood to go around. However, if you have type 2 diabetes, your liver never gets the memo instructing it to stop releasing glucose. It just keeps unloading the sweet stuff into the blood, forcing the pancreas to work overtime to crank out more insulin and making insulin's job of clearing sugar from the blood that much harder. Metformin takes some of the burden off the poor pancreas by fixing the problem with the liver; with less glucose hanging around in the blood, the demand for insulin drops. The medication is typically taken twice a day.

When metformin is used alone, it doesn't cause hypoglycemia. It is also less likely than some other diabetes medications to make you pack on pounds. Some metformin users even lose weight.

Still, metformin is not free of potential problems. About one-third of patients who take it develop gastrointestinal problems, including upset stomach, gas, diarrhea, and vomiting. (Such unpleasant tummy troubles could have something to do with the weight loss experienced by some metformin users.) Headaches and fatigue may occur, too. The good news is that these side effects usually fade within a few weeks of beginning treatment with metformin. Starting with small doses and gradually building up may also help to forestall unpleasant side effects. Taking metformin with meals can reduce stomach distress, too.

Metformin is often the first medication prescribed to treat type 2 diabetes. But it is not for everyone. The drug *should not* be used by:

- heavy drinkers
- those with kidney or liver disease
- anyone over 80 years of age, unless tests show that the liver and kidneys are still working hard
- people who have congestive heart failure or any other condition that interferes with circulation
- those with serious asthma or lung disease
- pregnant women
- children

One last word about metformin: It lowers levels of vitamin B12 in 10 to 30 percent of patients. However, taking calcium supplements may offset the drop, since the body needs the mineral to absorb vitamin B_{12}. If metformin has been prescribed for you, ask your doctor if you should take extra calcium, as well.

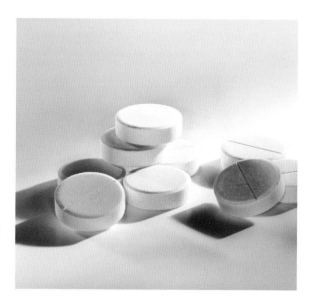

IS METFORMIN SAFE?

In a word, yes, though you may have heard that it causes a rare but deadly complication called lactic acidosis. Here's the reality: A predecessor of metformin, known as phenformin, was introduced in the 1950s. Phenformin worked like a charm, but it was banned in the United States in 1977 because some patients who took the drug developed lactic acidosis. Lactic acid is a waste product produced by cells when they burn glucose during hard exercise or other times when oxygen levels in the body are low. When too much lactic acid builds up, muscle pain, erratic heartbeat, rapid breathing, and other problems can result. Lactic acidosis is fatal about 40 percent of the time.

Scientists reconfigured the drug to eliminate the lactic acidosis threat, and Bristol-Myers Squibb introduced the new version, known as metformin, in 1995. Not surprisingly, doubts about the drug linger, and occasional reports arise of lactic acidosis in patients who take metformin. However, according to a commentary published in the July 2004 edition of *Diabetes Care*, an American Diabetes Association journal, virtually all cases of lactic acidosis linked to metformin have been in patients who took overdoses or shouldn't have been taking it in the first place, such as people with kidney disease or an excessive alcohol intake. According to the commentary, when metformin is used as labeled, the increased risk of lactic acidosis is either zero or very close to zero.

Sulfonylureas

Includes: chlorpropamide (Diabinese), glimepiride (Amaryl), glipizide (Glucotrol and Glucotrol XL), glyburide (Diabeta, Micronase) and micronized glyburide (Glynase)

Until this class of drugs was introduced in the 1950s, insulin was the only treatment available for people with diabetes. Sulfonylureas work by stimulating the beta cells in the pancreas to release more insulin into the bloodstream. They're usually taken once or twice a day before meals.

The sulfonylureas are usually broken down into older "first generation" pills and newer "second generation" pills. First generation sulfonylureas have fallen out of favor because, in general, the second-generation versions are more potent and have fewer side effects. Indeed, the only first-generation sulfonylurea still being used today is chlorpropamide. But the second generation isn't without its faults.

For example, these drugs, like the first-generation sulfonylureas, can cause hypoglycemia. A healthy pancreas is acutely sensitive to glucose levels in the blood, so it only produces as much insulin as the body needs. But sulfonylureas keep the beta cells working all the time, so a steady stream of insulin pours into the blood whether it's needed or not. As a result, blood sugar levels can drop too low, causing hypoglycemia. (This problem is especially common in the elderly and people who have liver or kidney disease.) On the other hand, if the prescribed dose of sulfonylurea is too low, the blood sugar can remain too high and continue to cause damage to the body. The prescribing physician can tinker with the dose to help relieve these problems, however.

Sulfonylureas can also cause weight gain as well as heartburn and other stomach problems. And drinking alcohol while taking certain sulfonylurea drugs may cause nausea, vomiting, and flushed skin.

Finally, sulfonylureas can sometimes lose their ability to control a person's blood sugar levels. Diabetes is a progressive disease, so over time, some of the insulin-producing beta cells in the pancreas will simply die off or slow down production. As beta-cell function decreases, the same amount of a sulfonylurea medication will be less effective at reducing glucose. When this occurs, the patient's doctor may prescribe another sulfonylurea instead or may simply drop the sulfonylurea altogether and switch the patient to another type of diabetes medication.

Meglitinides

Includes: nateglinide (Starlix), repaglinide (Prandin)
These drugs act like sulfonylureas that have

had too much caffeine. They are even sometimes referred to as nonsulfonylurea secretagogues because, like sulfonylureas, they trigger the beta cells of the pancreas to "secrete," or release, insulin. The difference is that meglitinides are impatient: They want that insulin released *now*. What's more, while sulfonylureas linger in the body all day, meglitinides rush in and out quickly. Because of their hyperactive nature, meglitinides play a specific role in managing type 2 diabetes: They are taken immediately before each of a day's three meals to boost insulin production in order to lower the predictable post-meal rise in blood sugar. (And if a meal is skipped, the dose of meglitinide is skipped as well.)

Meglitinides appear to cause hypoglycemia less often than sulfonylureas do, but it's still a possibility, especially if the dose is too high. Meglitinides can also cause weight gain. Other side effects are uncommon but can include backaches, headaches, cold and flu symptoms, chest pain, gastrointestinal problems, joint pain, tingling skin, certain infections, and vomiting.

Thiazolidinediones (Glitazones or TZDs)

Includes: pioglitazone (Actos), rosiglitazone (Avandia)
This group of medications is sometimes referred to as insulin sensitizers, which is a clue to how they work. Remember that in type 2 diabetes, problems begin with the condition known as insulin resistance. The pancreas does its job of releasing insulin, and the insulin tries

mightily to usher glucose into muscle and fat cells, but too often, the cells' insulin resistance prevents the hormone from succeeding. As a result, the pancreas must work harder to make more insulin in order for the cells to get the fuel they need. It's as though the cells can't hear insulin molecules knocking until there's a mob of them outside the door.

The glitazones make cells more sensitive to insulin so that they respond to a light tap on the door and allow glucose to enter. Of course, the actual way glitazones work is a bit more complex, but the bottom line is this: These drugs reduce insulin resistance, which helps keep blood sugar levels under control. The insulin-making beta cells of the pancreas, in turn, don't have to work so hard. That means they're less likely to conk out altogether and leave the body dependent on injections of insulin.

While the glitazones increase insulin sensitivity, they do not actually cause the body to make more of the hormone. Therefore, when used alone, glitazones do not cause low blood sugar.

The Food and Drug Administration (FDA) ordered an early version of these drugs, called troglitazone (under the brand name Rezulin), taken off the market in the United States in 2000. The problem: While troglitazone did a spiffy job of controlling blood sugar, in rare cases it caused serious—sometimes fatal—liver damage. The FDA declared that two other similar drugs, rosiglitazone and pioglitazone, were safer to use, although rosiglitazone

has been associated with liver abnormalities. If your doctor prescribes one of these two drugs, therefore, he or she will undoubtedly insist on monitoring your liver function through occasional blood tests.

The FDA also recently lifted restrictions on the use of rosiglitazone that it put in place back in 2010. Those restrictions were prompted by a different concern: short-term study results suggesting that the drug caused an increased risk of heart attack compared to metformin and sulfonylureas. In late 2013, however, the FDA removed most of those restrictions, stating that both a re-evaluation of the original research by outside experts as well as its own review of longer-term study data indicate that rosiglitazone is no more likely to cause a heart attack than the two standard types of diabetes medications. Still, the agency concedes that some "scientific uncertainty" about the cardio-vascular safety of rosiglitazone remains. So it's extremely important that people with type 2 diabetes work very closely with their physicians to determine if rosiglitazone's potential benefits outweigh its risks for them specifically before starting this drug.

As with many diabetes drugs, the glitazones may cause weight gain. Other possible side effects include headache, backache, muscle aches, fatigue, sinus inflammation, and swelling or fluid retention. This class of medication is not recommended for use during pregnancy. And female patients of childbearing age may need to take extra precautions if they don't want to get pregnant, because the glitazones can lower blood levels of oral contraceptives, making them less effective. Glitazones also appear to increase ovulation in some women, making them more fertile.

Alpha-Glucosidase Inhibitors (AGIs)

Includes: acarbose (Precose), miglitol (Glyset)

Alpha-glucosidase is a type of enzyme that lines the small intestine. Its job is to break down certain forms of sugar—starches, such as bread and potatoes, and sucrose, or table sugar—into glucose molecules small enough to pass into the bloodstream. Alpha-glucosidase inhibitors (AGIs) interfere with these enzymes, delaying the digestion and absorption of these sugars. These medications are taken with the first bite of food to help prevent post-meal sugar spikes. (If a meal is skipped, the dose of the AGI is skipped.)

AGIs are not without their faults, however. Have you ever eaten a bowl of baked beans or other similarly bean-laden dish, then experienced certain socially embarrassing side effects the next day? The same thing can happen with AGIs. Beans are packed with fiber, which your body can't digest. Like fiber, all the starch that is more slowly digested when you use an AGI eventually makes it to the large intestine, where it becomes fodder for the good bacteria normally living there. The process by which bacteria break down fiber, starch, or any other undigested sugar produces gas. The resulting flatulence, abdominal pain, and diarrhea can be bad enough that some patients plead with their doctors to give them a prescription for some other drug.

Some patients find that these problems with the body's food-processing apparatus aren't as severe if they start with a small dose.

AGIs don't cause hypoglycemia, although taking them with certain other diabetic drugs can produce low blood sugar. If hypoglycemia does develop during treatment with one of these drugs, certain sugary foods—the ones affected by AGIs—will not be effective in quickly bringing blood sugar back up to the normal range. Glucose tablets, honey, or fruit juice will still do the trick, however.

If you have had any serious intestinal condition in the past, your doctor probably won't recommend these drugs. Likewise, AGIs are usually considered off-limits for pregnant women.

DPP-4 Inhibitors

Includes: alogliptin (Nesina), linagliptin (Trajenta), saxagliptin (Onglyza), sitagliptan (Januvia)

This new class of oral diabetes medications helps to control blood sugar levels, particularly after meals. These drugs affect incretins, the hormones produced by the intestines that instruct the pancreas to make and release more insulin when you eat in order to keep the blood sugar levels from skyrocketing. One of the most important of these incretins is GLP-1. GLP-1 also aids blood sugar control by decreasing the amount of the hormone glucagon that the pancreas sends to the liver near mealtimes. Normally, an enzyme in the body called DPP-4 quickly turns off GLP-1 and the other incretins. The DPP-4 inhibitor medications block this enzyme, allowing GLP-1 to do a better job of keeping blood sugar levels in check.

Non-Insulin Injectable Drugs

In recent years, scientists have developed some promising new diabetes drugs that do not contain insulin but still must be injected. No, the developers weren't trying to be mean by opting for the injectable form. These drugs simply must be injected in order to bypass the stomach and enter the bloodstream directly. And the tiny needle stick is worth the payoff—better glucose control.

DPP-4 Inhibitors are typically taken once a day, at the same time each day. They can be taken alone or in combination with other diabetes medications. When used alone, they do not cause low blood sugar. And while they don't help with weight loss, they also don't cause weight gain, as several other diabetes medications can. Reported side effects of DPP-4 inhibitors include stuffy nose, sore throat, and upper respiratory infection; headache; and digestive discomforts such as diarrhea and abdominal pain.

Incretin Mimetics
Includes: exenatide (Byetta), Liraglutide (Victoza)
The Gila monster is a brawny, two-foot-long lizard with a brutal, venomous bite that lives in the desert of the southwestern United States. Why the zoology lesson? Because this scaly critter produces a hormone that may be the key to better glucose control for some people with type 2 diabetes.

Here's the reason: The Gila monster only eats four times a year—mostly small animals, eggs, and whatever else it can find. The rest of the year, the big lizard survives off fat packed away in its chunky tail and belly. Since it would be pointless, and probably not too healthy, to keep cranking out insulin during those long months between meals, the Gila monster's body evolved the ability to turn off its pancreas. That led researchers to wonder: When a Gila monster finally does sit down to dinner, it needs insulin to process food. How does it turn its pancreas back on? Scientists eventually discovered a hormone called exendin-4 in the Gila monster's saliva, of all places. To be more precise, exendin-4 is an incretin hormone that's produced in the intestines. Humans make incretins, too. When you eat, your gut senses glucose and imme-diately sends incretins to the pancreas with orders to produce insulin. But in people with type 2 diabetes, the signal from incretins is too weak to stimulate insulin production.

Exendin-4, on the other hand, has to be potent enough to arouse a pancreas that's been snoozing for months. The injectable diabetes drug exenatide is a synthetic version of exendin-4. Because exenatide imitates (or "mimes") exendin-4, it's called an incretin mimetic.

Studies show that exenatide keeps blood sugar low not only by stimulating insulin production but also by instructing the pancreas to make less of that other critical hormone, glucagon. As glucagon is suppressed, the liver in turn puts out less glucose. That means less strain on the pancreas. In fact, some research suggests that exenatide even causes the pancreas to make new insulin-producing beta cells in the pancreas.

Exenatide also causes food to pass through your stomach at a more leisurely rate, which slows the typically rapid rise in glucose after a meal. It also means your belly feels full longer, so you eat less. In fact, while most diabetes drugs cause weight gain, exenatide seems to have the opposite effect. In one study, people with type 2 diabetes who took the drug for 30 weeks lost more than six pounds, on average.

So what's the catch? Although it's a power-ful drug, exenatide is rather delicate in one sense: It can't tolerate the rough trip through your gastrointestinal system, so it has to be injected just like insulin. Exenatide doses come in prepackaged "pens," similar to the ones used by many diabetes patients who require insulin injections. Exenatide users give them-selves two injections per day, before breakfast and dinner. Because most people would rather swallow a pill than stick a needle into their belly or backside, doctors may not prescribe exenatide unless other oral diabetes pills fail to keep a patient's glucose under control.

Exenatide can cause nausea, though it often fades over time. Some other side effects that users have reported include vomiting, diarrhea, the jitters, dizziness, headaches, and

upset stomach. Taken alone, exenatide doesn't cause hypoglycemia, but blood sugar may drop too low if the drug is paired with one of the sulfonylureas. People who have kidney disease or serious gastrointestinal problems shouldn't use exenatide. Animal studies show that exenatide may harm fetuses, so women who use the drug and become pregnant may be switched to another medication.

Amylin Mimetics

Includes: pramlintide (Symlin)

Let's get the unwelcome news out of the way first: Like exenatide, pramlintide is an injected drug. Then again, if your doctor prescribes pramlintide, you are probably already used to pricking and poking yourself, since the medication is used in conjunction with insulin injections. That means folks with type 1 diabetes as well as those with type 2 can use it.

Pramlintide is a synthetic version of yet another hormone that plays an important role in controlling blood sugar. It turns out that the beta cells in the pancreas hold down two jobs. Not only do they produce insulin, they also make the hormone amylin. Beta cells churn out amylin at the same time as insulin when we eat. Like the incretins discussed previously, amylin lowers glucagon levels, so the liver doesn't release unneeded glucose. It also makes the stomach empty into the intestines more slowly after a meal, which prevents glucose spikes.

Unfortunately, if you have type 2 diabetes, your beta cells may be so beat up that you're not producing enough amylin. If you have type 1 diabetes, you probably aren't making the hormone at all. By replacing amylin, therefore, pramlintide helps keep blood sugar levels stable after meals. Some users even lose a few pounds. Your doctor will only add pramlintide to your daily regimen if insulin injections have failed to lower your glucose levels into the safe zone.

Pramlintide is injected just like insulin at mealtimes. But the two hormones don't blend well, so you can't combine the two drugs into one syringe. If you need to take both drugs, you'll still have to inject twice.

Monitoring your blood sugar is a must if you're using pramlintide (as it is if you're injecting insulin); if your blood sugar is a bit on the low side, a dose of the drug could send it into a freefall and you'll develop severe hypoglycemia. The most common side effect of pramlintide is nausea, followed by loss of appetite, headache, vomiting, stomach pain, fatigue, dizziness, and upset stomach. You might also develop redness, pain, or minor bruising at the spot where you inject pramlintide.

It's also important to talk to your doctor about any other medications you may be taking if he or she prescribes pramlintide. Because it slows down activity in your stomach, pramlintide could alter the effectiveness of some drugs.

Insulin Therapy

When doctors abandoned the old name "non-insulin-dependent diabetes mellitus" in favor of the sleeker "type 2 diabetes," they weren't merely opting for a time-saving moniker. They were acknowledging that, for at least one-quarter of their patients with the condition, the old name is just plain wrong. Although most people with type 2 diabetes have a functioning pancreas when first diagnosed, over time their beta cells may not be able to keep up with demand for insulin, even if oral or non-insulin injectable diabetes drugs are added to diet and exercise therapy.

Research shows that oral medications are frequently not enough for patients to maintain healthy blood sugar. For instance, a 1998 British study of nearly 600 people with type 2 diabetes found that within three years of starting on metformin and a sulfonylurea, just one-third of patients had A1c readings below 7 percent. This is critical, as over the long term, levels higher than 7 percent can lead to organ damage. On the other hand, properly executed insulin therapy is just about foolproof, with a stellar track record for lowering blood sugar.

When blood tests reveal glucose levels that remain stubbornly high, doctors will usually advise insulin therapy. Although many physicians once considered insulin injections to be the treatment of last resort for their patients with type 2 diabetes, many now see this form of hormone replacement therapy as a way to better manage the disease at earlier stages in order to prevent the serious, debilitating complications that can result from chronically elevated blood sugar.

THE INS AND OUTS
OF INSULIN THERAPY

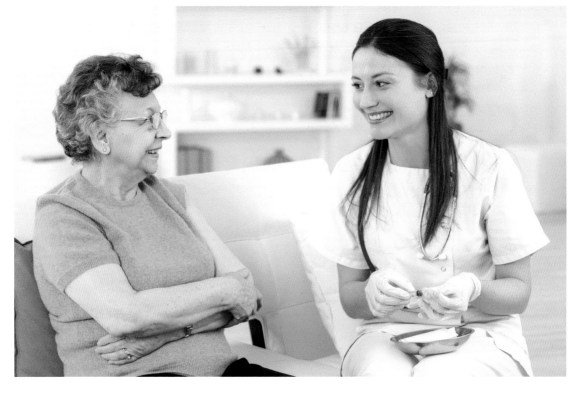

People with type 1 diabetes are well aware of the value of insulin therapy. After all, without the hormone injections, they would die. For folks with type 2 diabetes who have been advised to begin insulin injections, however, fear, misinformation, or uncertainty can keep them from seeing—and taking advantage of—the therapy's very real benefits.

Overcome Your Fear

When a patient with type 2 diabetes can no longer control blood sugar with diet, exercise, and oral medication, the next obvious step is to begin insulin therapy. However, doctors say that many patients have an emotional response to this news and resist the idea of taking insulin. Indeed, some patients bring a whole new meaning to the phrase "insulin resistance" when their physicians bring up the therapy. They may refuse the treatments because they don't believe they can administer them properly. Or they want nothing to do with needles. Or maybe they associate insulin therapy with their old Aunt Mabel who took the injections but still went blind or ended up in a wheelchair.

When a patient is hesitant or flat-out refuses to take insulin, physicians sometimes say he or she has psychological insulin resistance, or PIR. Several studies reflect the prevalence of PIR. In one large trial, more than one-quarter of type 2 patients who were prescribed insulin refused to take the drug, at least initially. In another study, up to three-quarters of patients said they were reluctant to take insulin. But the longer such therapy is put off, the more damage high blood sugar has a chance to do.

Two experts on diabetes and behavior— William H. Polonsky, Ph.D., of the University of California–San Diego, and Richard A. Jackson, M.D., of Boston's Joslin Diabetes Center—have identified six attitudes and beliefs that can cause PIR. Here they are, followed by a healthy dose of reality:

1. Patients view taking insulin as a loss of control. In one survey, half of patients interviewed said they believed that insulin therapy would restrict or disrupt their lives. Some patients worry that taking insulin will rob their lives of spontaneity, make travel and dining out difficult, and create other hassles. Others worry about the threat of hypoglycemia and weight gain.

The facts: The wide variety of insulin available can accommodate most lifestyles and allow for spur-of-the-moment changes in plans. Yes, hypoglycemia is a concern, but once a patient learns to manage insulin therapy and oral medications, it is a less common occurrence. Weight gain caused by insulin, if any, is usually modest.

2. Patients lack confidence in their ability. Giving yourself insulin injections is definitely trickier than popping a pill once or twice a day. Not surprisingly, nearly half of patients prescribed insulin worry that they will make mistakes by messing up the timing or delivering the wrong dosage. Unfortunately, self-doubt can turn into a self-fulfilling prophesy, as patients who lack confidence often do a poor of job managing insulin treatments.

The facts: Worries about proper technique can be overcome by working closely with your diabetes educator and—as the old saying goes—practice, practice, practice. Using an insulin pen instead of a needle may be less intimidating.

3. Patients feel a sense of failure. Patients often say that needing insulin is proof that they did a poor job of taking care of their diabetes. As Polonsky and Jackson explain, "insulin is viewed as a well-deserved punishment for one's own gluttony, sloth, or negligence . . ."

The facts: Diabetes is a chronic disease, and many patients eventually require additional forms of treatment, including insulin therapy. Accepting that possibility early on can eliminate the shock factor if the need arises.

4. Patients have misconceptions about insulin. A patient will often see a prescription for insulin as proof that his or her condition is worsening. Moreover, some patients worry that insulin itself makes you sick. That may be especially true if an older relative lost eyesight or required amputation soon after beginning insulin treatments.

The facts: While taking insulin slightly increases the risk of hypoglycemia, there is no truth to myths such as "insulin makes you go blind." When a patient's condition worsens soon after commencing insulin therapy, it's likely that years of poorly controlled blood sugar were the culprit.

5. Some patients have needle phobia. Many patients complain that they don't want—or won't have the guts—to jab themselves with a sharp object several times a day for the rest of their lives.

The facts: A mental health counselor can help patients overcome fear of needles. Genuine needle phobia is relatively uncommon. In many cases, patients discover that their anxiety about injecting themselves comes from their frustration with having diabetes.

6. Patients often have "What's In It for Me?" syndrome. A patient who is overcome with doubts and fears about insulin may have a hard time believing the drug's benefits outweigh perceived potential harm. One study found that only one in ten type 2 diabetes patients believed that insulin therapy would improve their health.

The facts: Attaining better glucose control through insulin therapy not only reduces the risk for long-term complications, it can also improve mood, energy level, and sleep quality.

What Type of Insulin Should You Use?

If you are currently taking oral diabetes drugs and your doctor wants to add insulin to your regimen, there are several different varieties to choose from. Some hit your bloodstream and start working right away, while others take their time and last all day. This section provides an overview of the types of insulin available.

In the early days of insulin therapy, there was only one variety. After the hormone was injected, it started lowering glucose levels in 60 minutes or less, reached its peak performance within a few hours, and then fizzled out, lasting no longer than eight hours. This type, known simply as regular insulin, is still used in diabetes management today.

Scientists eventually figured out that tweaking the amino acids (the building blocks of proteins) in insulin made it behave differently. In particular, they were able to alter the speed at which insulin is absorbed by the body. The longer it takes your body to absorb a drug, the longer it remains active. This discovery has led to a wider variety of insulin choices that can help you and your doctor tailor your insulin injections to your body's needs.

By tinkering with insulin's molecules, scientists can have been able to alter insulin's speed and durability in three ways:

- **Onset:** how long it takes the insulin to enter your bloodstream and get to work lowering your blood glucose
- **Peak time:** how long it takes insulin to reach maximum strength, when it works hardest
- **Duration:** how long the insulin works before it quits

All this variety adds up to several benefits for you. For starters, longer-acting insulin can reduce the number of injections you need in a day. What's more, combining two different types of insulin may help improve glucose control. For example, your doctor might prescribe a long-acting form of insulin called glargine, which has no peak but stays active for 24 hours, slowly letting insulin into your system to maintain daily business. But to accommodate the spike of glucose that hits your system after eating, you may also take a premeal blast of short-acting insulin. Ultimately, the goal is to create a hormonal environment in your body that mimics what your pancreas would do, if only it could.

Premixed insulin represents an option for patients who take two different types of insulin. There are a number of premeasured preparations available that typically blend short- and long-acting forms of insulin or intermediate- and short-acting forms. The goal of using premixed insulin is to reduce the number of injections the patient must make in a day. Premixed insulin has some benefits and downsides, so it isn't for everyone.

Advantages of premixed insulin:
- no need to play chemist, since the insulin is mixed for you
- fewer daily injections

Disadvantages of premixed insulin:
- premixed solutions require you to eat a specific amount of food at set times and to strictly adhere to a regular schedule of physical activity
- harder to maintain normal glucose control

Tools for Injecting Insulin

Wouldn't it be swell if insulin came in an easy-to-swallow pill or maybe a tasty beverage? Unfortunately, tiny, sensitive insulin molecules wouldn't stand a chance in the hostile environs of your stomach, where digestive enzymes would rip them to shreds. That means you have to bypass your gut and deliver this must-have hormone directly into your bloodstream. Traditionally, that has required an injection through the skin.

Hypodermic Syringes

Just reading those words can make you wince. Your doctor has been jabbing you with these sharp objects since you were a tiny tot. Syringes are cylinders with plungers on one end and hollow needles fitted into the other. Fortunately, the needles used to inject insulin have gone on a crash diet in recent years. They're sharper than ever, too. Slender gauges and finer points mean they hurt less. Some have special slick coatings, too, which let the needle slide under your skin more easily. Anyone who takes insulin will tell you that it's a bigger deal to test your blood glucose than to give yourself a shot. Your doctor or diabetes educator will help you select a syringe that's appropriate for the dose of insulin you'll be taking.

Insulin "Pens"

Warning: These insulin tools really do look like writing instruments, so don't accidentally take out your fountain pen and give yourself a dose of India ink. Like the implements you use for writing, some insulin pens use replaceable cartridges and are designed for long-term use; others are disposable (you toss them out after the prefilled pen is empty).

Insulin pens allow you to "dial" the dose of insulin you need. You simply place the tip to your skin and press the plunger to inject. Speaking of tips, here's a good one: When injecting insulin with a pen, count to six slowly before pulling out the needle in order to keep insulin from leaking out of the injection site. (The same advice applies to short syringe needles.) Some people find insulin pens more convenient, especially if they have to inject frequently. What's more, people who use other methods for injecting insulin (such as syringes or pumps) often carry an insulin pen as an emergency backup.

Jet Injectors

Got a bad case of belonephobia? That's the medical term for fear of needles and other sharp objects. You're in good company; about one person in ten is needle-phobic. An insulin jet injector may be just what you need. These clever tools use high pressure to force a jet stream of insulin through the skin. There is a possible downside, though: Jet injectors can cause bruising.

Insulin Pumps

Short of an organ transplant, an insulin pump is the closest thing to a full-time replacement for a pooped-out pancreas. An insulin pump is a small battery-operated computer, about the size of a pager. (This is a big improvement over the original model introduced in the 1970s, which was strapped onto the patient's back like some sort of jet pack.) The computer is attached to a flexible tube with a catheter on the tip. The computer contains an insulin reservoir, and it clips onto a belt, waistband, or some other article of clothing. Using an insertion needle, you place the catheter just under the skin, usually on the abdomen. The process is similar to giving yourself a standard insulin injection, with a big exception: Once you have inserted the catheter, it can remain in place for two or three days before it needs to be replaced and the injection site changed (to prevent infection). And you know what that means—fewer needle jabs.

Based on how much insulin you need and the type you use, you program the computer to deliver an even dose of the hormone (known as basal insulin) throughout the day. However, for greater flexibility, you can override the computer program with the press of a button and give yourself little pick-me-up doses (called bolus insulin) when necessary, such as immediately before eating. And maybe after eating, too, if you had not planned to have dessert but your willpower crumbled when the waiter uttered the words "chocolate cheesecake." It's easy enough to compensate for the occasional splurge. Some pump manufacturers have even integrated continous glucose monitoring into their devices, so that users don't have to separately test their blood sugar and punch in their results multiple times a day. Plus, the more exact control the pump provides helps prevent hypoglycemia, which can lead to weight gain when extra glucose must be consumed to raise a blood sugar level that's been lowered too far by too much insulin. Studies suggest that people with diabetes who use insulin pumps are better able to manage their blood sugar levels than those who use other methods. That improved management, in turn, can translate into fewer diabetes complications.

Pumps do have a few potential disadvantages, however. Infection is a risk if you don't change the insertion site frequently or get sloppy with your technique. Also, mechanical problems can cause a pump to malfunction, and tubes may become jammed. Or you could simply run out of insulin and not realize it. Any one of these problems could cause glucose levels to soar,

resulting in a life-threatening condition called ketoacidosis. However, improvements in pump technology make these problems rare.

Insulin pumps are pricey, too—typically in the four figures; however, most health insurers (including Medicare and Medicaid) will cover at least some of the cost.

Perhaps the most obvious problem with insulin pumps is figuring out what to do with the tiny computer when you exercise, sleep, go skinny-dipping, or engage in any other activity where you might find it inconvenient to have an electronic appliance attached to your belly. Most devices, however, can be temporarily disconnected from the injection site so that they won't get in the way or be damaged during such activities.

Despite these potential issues, it's pretty clear that people with diabetes who try the insulin pump find these minor hassles worth tolerating and like the convenience of a device that frees them from making scheduled injections. After all, the insulin pump's popularity rises every year. According to the journal *Postgraduate Medicine*, the number of users in the United States rose from just 6,000 in 1990 to 162,000 by 2001. By 2004, the number of users was estimated at 200,000, and today it's somewhere near 350,000, according to *Diabetes Self-Management*. The magazine further notes that roughly 30,000 of those 350,000 diabetic pump users are thought to have type 2.

in Inhalers

:utical companies have long sought a painfree way to administer insulin, certain that such an invention would be instantly popular among people with diabetes who otherwise have to (or have been advised to) inject the hormone with needles. In mid 2006, the drug maker Pfizer received Food and Drug Administration (FDA) approval to introduce Exubera, the first major alternative to needle injections since the discovery of insulin. Exubera was a form of powdered insulin that patients inhaled through a plastic handheld device similar to the inhalers that are used by people with asthma and allergies. Diabetes patients could use Exubera instead of injecting rapid-acting insulin before meals. Yet the drug didn't catch on, and after less than two years on the market, poor sales forced Pfizer to discontinue the product. Those dismal results also prompted two other drug companies to halt the inhaled-insulin products they had in the works. At least part of the reason that Exubera failed could be traced to the fact that insurers refused to pay for it, saying it was too expensive compared to the standard needle-based delivery systems and that it wasn't effective for many people with diabetes.

Considering the obvious appeal of a needle-less insulin delivery system, however, it's not surprising that another company is once again introducing an insulin inhalation sys-tem. The California-based company MannKind has worked with the FDA since 2009 to gain approval for its inhaled insulin powder, which it calls Afrezza. The inhalation device, called Dreamboat, is considerably smaller than the Exubera device: Roughly the size of a child's toy whistle, it fits easily in the palm of the hand. But Afrezza's greatest appeal may be in how quickly and how well it works in people with either type 1 or type 2 diabetes.

Recent research indicates that Afrezza is actually more effective than oral diabetes drugs and injectable insulins in matching the way the body's own natural insulin works. When inhaled as the Afrezza powder, the insulin reaches peak levels in 12 to 14 minutes—in other words, in the same amount of time that the body's own insulin peaks in a person who does not have diabetes.

The research further indicates that Afrezza is effective at lowering blood sugar levels in the long term, as measured by A1c testing. And MannKind has said that the cost of its drug could be roughly equivalent to the cost of using one of the insulin pens already on the market.

As with the previous inhaled insulin product, Afrezza may not be appropriate for certain people. If you have asthma or lung disease, for example, or if you smoke, chances are the drug will be off-limits to you. And inhaled formulations in the past were known to some-times cause a cough or at least a slight loss of lung function.

But if you think you might be interested in this type of insulin delivery system, talk to your doctor about it.

AVOIDING HIGHS AND LOWS

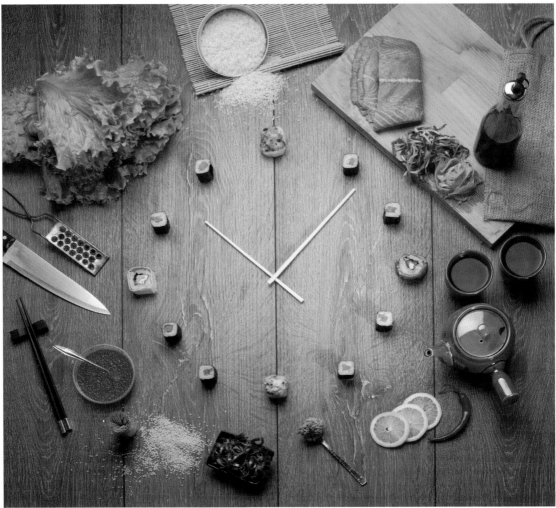

In many aspects of life, success depends on finding the right balance. Likewise, the key challenge in managing diabetes is keeping your blood sugar in a happy state of equilibrium. Yet, there are many ways to disrupt this balance, including—ironically—taking the very medications you may use to control diabetes. Knowing how to recognize and respond to the symptoms of high and low blood sugar will help is crucial.

Hypoglycemia: The Basics

Keeping blood sugar from rising too high is the goal for anyone with any variety of diabetes. But hypoglycemia is, in a sense, the result of too much success. When glucose levels drop off, cells throughout much of the body can adjust by living off fat and protein, at least temporarily. But one very important organ—the one located between your ears—can't use fat and protein for energy. Since the brain needs glucose to survive, it regards a sugar shortage as a crisis. Early symptoms are no big deal. You feel hungry and a little shaky and nervous, like you had too much coffee. But soon you begin to feel woozy and need to sit down. Your heart thumps, and you break into a cold sweat. Unless you take the proper steps, you may become confused and talk incoherently. Your vision blurs and your head feels ready to burst. In extreme cases, hypoglycemia causes convulsions and even comas.

What causes a plunge in blood sugar? In a person who does not have diabetes, hypoglycemia is fairly uncommon. When blood sugar begins to drop, the pancreas senses trouble and slows down insulin production, so the body doesn't use up glucose so quickly. For an added boost, the pancreas makes the hormone glucagon, which signals the liver to convert some glycogen (the storage form of sugar) to glucose, then release the sugary stuff into the blood.

But this system can get out of whack if you have diabetes, making it tricky to maintain balanced blood sugar. That's especially true if you inject insulin or take a sulfonylurea or meglitinide, two widely used types of oral medication that perk up insulin production in the pancreas. Getting the proper dose of these therapies exactly right is something of an art. To avoid frequent bouts of hypoglycemia, you must become expert at tweaking your dosage.

Preventing Hypoglycemia

Chances are, you are going to experience at least a touch of hypoglycemia now and then. Accepting that these occasional spells are part of coping with diabetes can make them less upsetting or disruptive. Better yet, take the following advice and limit your bouts with low blood sugar.

Medications

Insulin therapy and insulin-stimulating drugs are lifesavers. But these treatments know how to do one thing—lower blood sugar. Even when glucose levels reach perilously low levels, they keep doing just that, ignoring cues from the body to knock it off. One common cause of hypoglycemia is medication overkill: Even though you took the recommended dose, it was more medicine than your body needed.

In other words, you artificially increased insulin levels beyond the amount you needed to control blood sugar. This can occur because you took too much medicine, of course. But often this problem is unavoidable and happens even if you do everything right. Your quirky corpus can change its mind about how much insulin it needs from day to day. You can even monitor your glucose levels with the vigilance of a hawk and still end up having a hypoglycemic episode. However, various lifestyle decisions and choices you make every day will affect how well insulin therapies work.

Meals

Say you are about to head down to the cafeteria for lunch when the boss asks if you faxed that 50-page document to Los Angeles—the one that was supposed to be there an hour ago. Or you're halfway through dinner when your long-lost twin sister Mildred shows up at the door. You are probably not going to say, "Great to see you, Millie, but give me five minutes while I finish this tuna sandwich."

Because you have diabetes, you must be sure that your body has enough insulin to process the food you eat, especially if you inject insulin or take sulfonylureas or meglitinides. But when you skip or put off a meal—or eat less than you planned—you can end up with more insulin than you need.

Tips

- Try to eat meals and snacks at the same time every day.
- Avoid skipping meals.
- Clean your plate—eat as much as you planned. However, if you find that you need to overeat in order to prevent low blood glucose, discuss this with your doctor.
- Talk to your doctor or diabetes educator about what to do on days when interruptions to your meal routine are unavoidable.

Exercise and Other Physical Activity

Keeping fit has unquestionable benefits for anyone with diabetes. But if you have diabetes, especially the type 1 variety, exercise requires a bit more planning. The problem begins with your muscles. During exertion, their fuel demand skyrockets. In a person who does not have diabetes, insulin levels drop and glucagon rises, causing the liver to release glucose so cells can burn it as energy. As a result, blood sugar levels remain fairly constant.

Unfortunately, if you have type 1 diabetes, your pancreas doesn't respond to exercise and the greater demand for glucose by reducing insulin levels because, well, you don't have any insulin to cut back on. Instead, you add insulin to your blood by injecting it. But the dose you need while sitting around the house staring at the fish tank is much higher than what you need while playing full-court basketball. If you don't adjust the dose accordingly, high insulin levels in the blood will prevent your liver from releasing stored glucose and, as a result, your blood sugar levels will fall.

Exercise-induced hypoglycemia is also a concern for people with type 2 diabetes who take a sulfonylurea or meglitinide. Although your pancreas may want to slow insulin production during exercise, both drugs make sure it continues to pump out the hormone.

Beware another postworkout phenomenon known as delayed hypoglycemia. After exercising, your tired muscles restock themselves with glucose and your liver takes its sweet time re-building its inventory of glycogen (the stored form of glucose). While all this is going on, blood sugar can remain low. If you don't eat enough food after strenuous exercise, delayed hypoglycemia can strike—usually between 6 and 15 hours later. But delayed hypoglycemia can actually occur as many as 28 hours after a workout. One study found that over a two-year period, 48 out of approximately 300 young type 1 diabetes patients had a bout with delayed hypoglycemia. The problem may be more likely to occur if you work out more intensely than usual.

Tips

- Talk with your doctor or diabetes educa-tor about adjusting your insulin dose or your snack intake before working out, playing a sport, or participating in any other physical activity that will make you huff and puff.

- Inject insulin in the abdomen before exercise; research shows that flexing, stretching, pumping limb muscles absorb injected insulin too quickly during exercise.

- Plan on having a snack during very long bouts of exercise, such as long-distance running or cross-coun-try skiing.

- Consider eating a snack after a long workout to help reduce the risk for de-layed hypoglycemia.

- Monitor, monitor, monitor. Check your blood sugar levels before and after exercising—even during, if you're in the gym or on the track for a long time.

Alcohol

If you know a little about the chemistry of alcoholic beverages, it may seem odd to learn that drinking booze can cause low blood sugar. After all, many forms of alcohol con-tain carbohydrates. In fact, if you are well fed, drinking a lot of alcohol can have the opposite effect, causing blood sugar to soar too high. However, drinking alcohol on an empty stom-ach can cause your blood sugar to plummet. If you haven't eaten in a while, your blood sugar levels may already be on the low side. Without food to break down into glucose, your liver converts stored glycogen into simple sugar, which it releases into the blood to keep your organs functioning, especially your brain.

But tossing back a few cocktails or glasses of wine when your body is relying on the liver for its supply of glucose can turn happy hour into a horror show. Alcohol interferes with the liver's ability to produce glucose molecules, which can leave the body bereft of its most efficient energy source.

Sweet Salvation: Treating Hypoglycemia

If you have diabetes and suddenly notice that you feel light-headed and jittery, especially if you use insulin therapy, there's an excellent chance you have developed hypoglycemia. But confirming your suspicion is a good idea, since low blood sugar can occur for other reasons.

Here's yet another good reason to keep your glucose meter handy. If a spot check reveals a glucose reading that's 70 mg/dl or lower, low blood sugar is the culprit.

The solution is surprisingly straightforward. You don't have to take a special drug that triggers your pancreas to produce hormones or that knocks out enzymes responsible for modulating some complex biochemical reaction. Your blood sugar is low, so the goal is to put more into circulation, ASAP. The fastest way to boost glucose is by consuming 15 grams of simple sugars, which break down rapidly in the body. You might have to give yourself another dose if your symptoms don't fade within 15 minutes or so.

Some good choices for boosting low blood sugar include:

- 2 or 3 glucose tablets
- ½ cup of fruit juice
- ½ cup of a regular soft drink (not a diet beverage, which contains no sugar)
- 1 cup of milk
- Small boxes of raisins
- 5 or 6 pieces of hard candy
- 1 or 2 teaspoons of honey or sugar
- A tube of glucose gel or other antihypoglycemia product

Other Causes of Hypoglycemia

Using insulin or insulin-stimulating medications increases the risk for low blood sugar,

but the problem can be triggered by other conditions and circumstances. If you develop symptoms but your glucose levels appear to be safe (and you know your glucose meter is working properly), talk to your doctor. Hypoglycemia can also be caused by:

- other medications, including aspirin, sulfa drugs (for treating infections), pentamidine (for serious pneumonia), and quinine (for malaria).

- alcohol, especially if you go on a bender. Heavy doses of booze interfere with the liver's ability to release glucose.

- other illnesses, including diseases of the heart, kidneys, and liver. Also, rare tumors called insulinomas produce insulin, which would raise levels of the hormone too high, causing blood sugar to drop.

- hormonal deficiencies. More common in children, a shortage of glucagon, as well as other hormones (including cortisol, growth hormone, and epinephrine) can cause hypoglycemia.

Hyperglycemia

Astute readers have probably already figured out that if hypoglycemia means too little glucose in the blood, then hyperglycemia must mean too much blood sugar. But isn't that the topic of this entire book? Isn't the basic problem of diabetes that you have too much sugar in your blood?

Yes, but the story is a bit more complex. Technically speaking, a doctor could say you have hyperglycemia if a blood test shows that your glucose is higher than it should be (usually defined as more than 100 mg/dl between meals and 140 mg/dl or higher after eating). It's no big deal if your glucose creeps up a little now and then, but chronically elevated blood sugar can be debilitating and potentially fatal.

But the term hyperglycemia can also refer to an acute case of very high blood sugar, which you definitely want to avoid, too. Hyperglycemia can lead to two serious conditions. One occurs primarily (though not exclusively) in people with type 1 diabetes, while the other is mostly a concern for type 2 patients.

Diabetic Ketoacidosis

You've learned about ketones, which are leftover products your body makes when it burns fat instead of glucose for energy. Any time you shed flab on a weight-loss diet, your body cranks out ketones. Still, your cells get some glucose on low-carb diets. In a person who does not have type 1 diabetes—whose pancreas still makes insulin—the concentration of ketones in your body while eating a low-carb diet never poses a serious health threat. However, trouble starts if your blood becomes flooded with ketones, which can happen if your body runs very low on insulin. That risk is always a possibility with type 1 diabetes. At first you may simply need to urinate a lot to unload all the glucose you're not burning. Since you're losing so much water in the urine, you'll become thirsty, too. As your blood becomes more saturated with ketones, you will probably begin to feel lousy in all ways—tired, nauseated, feverish. Your heart will race, and you'll pant like a big dog on a hot day. If you don't receive medical attention, you could slip into a coma and die.

Some common causes of diabetic ketoacidosis include:

- Infections. As your body fights bacteria, it produces hormones that interfere with insulin and trigger the liver to release glucose. Urinary tract infections are a common cause of ketoacidosis in patients with type 1 diabetes.

- Stress. Emotions can trigger a similar hormonal onslaught. The same is true of anything that stresses your body, such as trauma, a serious illness, or surgery.

- The "Oops" factor. As in, "Oops, I forgot to inject insulin before lunch." (Physicians favor the term "noncompliance.")

- Other insulin problems. Patients who use insulin pumps may not notice if the device becomes clogged or for some other reason fails to deliver a scheduled dose, and ketoacidosis could result. Injecting outdated insulin could have the same effect.

- The "I've Got What?" factor. Did those early symptoms of ketoacidosis—the unslakeable thirst, the well-worn path to the restroom—sound familiar? They should, since they are the early signs of type 1 diabetes. In fact, some patients learn for the first time that they have the disease when they develop ketoacidosis and see a doctor for treatment.

Preventing ketoacidosis is as simple as taking a quick trip to the bathroom or doing an additional fingerstick. A urine or blood ketone test can pick up signs of ketoacidosis before the symptoms get out of control. As a rule, it's a good idea to give yourself a ketone test if:

- your blood sugar is higher than 240 mg/dl (some doctors say 300 mg/dl is a better benchmark; ask your physician)

- you become nauseated or start vomiting

- you develop the flu, pneumonia, or any other serious illness

- you are pregnant

Talk to your doctor or diabetes educator about using urine ketone tests to detect ketoacidosis. Specifically, ask how often and when you should check for ketones and what you should do if a test turns up high levels.

Hyperosmolar Hyperglycemic Syndrome (HHS)

Despite the name, this condition has nothing to do with your molars. Instead, hyperosmolar hyperglycemic syndrome (HHS for short) occurs for lack of one of the most common elements—the clear, wet stuff that comes out of the tap in your kitchen or in overpriced bottles at the grocery store. Water is a critical player when glucose builds up in the blood. Normally, when blood sugar rises, the kidneys swing into action and lower levels by excreting excess glucose in the urine. But when the body's water supply runs low, the kidneys slow down urine production. Glucose builds up even more, further increasing demand for water.

Some of the symptoms of HHS resemble those of diabetic ketoacidosis, such as increased thirst, fatigue, and weakness. (HHS does not, however, produce paint-thinner breath, since it doesn't cause ketones to flood the blood.) As HHS progresses, patients may develop rapid heartbeat and sunken eyeballs. They may also become confused and move awkwardly. At advanced stages, HHS can lead to convulsions and coma.

In some cases, a glass of water is all it would take to prevent HHS. The condition often strikes elderly patients with type 2 diabetes (HHS is rare in type 1 patients) who become dehydrated because they can't tend to their own thirst or because whoever should be helping them to wet their whistles (nursing home attendants, for example) aren't getting the job done. Some other causes of HHS include:

- poorly treated or undiagnosed type 2 diabetes
- weak kidneys or kidney dialysis
- infections, heart attacks, and strokes—or any other stress on the body, such as surgery
- medications (Certain drugs used to treat

hypertension, asthma, and allergies can cause dehydration, block insulin, or raise glucose.)

- vomiting (Losing your lunch causes dehydration.)

HHS is definitely a medical emergency. Doctors treat the condition with intravenous fluids to rehydrate the body and insulin to bring down soaring glucose levels. However, patients have often lapsed into a coma by the time they arrive in an emergency room. HHS is fatal in up to 40 percent of cases. As with diabetic acidosis, the key to preventing HHS is vigilant monitoring—in this case with a glucose meter. If levels rise and don't come down, for any reason, contact your physician.

KNOW THE SIGNS OF LOW BLOOD SUGAR

Hypoglycemia, or low blood sugar, is a risk for anyone who has diabetes. However, it's most common among patients who inject insulin or take insulin-stimulating drugs, including sulfonylureas and meglitinides. Consider hypoglycemia when you begin to feel any of these symptoms:

- excessive hunger
- nervousness
- the jitters or shakiness
- sweating for no apparent reason
- anxiety
- weakness, loss of coordination
- dizziness or feeling light-headed
- unusual sleepiness
- confusion
- difficulty speaking
- blurred vision

If any of the following occurs while you're in bed, low blood sugar is a possibility:

- You have a nightmare or cry out in your sleep.
- You awaken with your pajamas or bed sheets soaked with perspiration. (Even if there's a chance that your night sweats could be associated with perimenopause, play it safe and check your blood glucose level.)
- In the morning you feel tired, confused, or irritable or you awaken with a headache.

PROTECTING AND PREVENTING

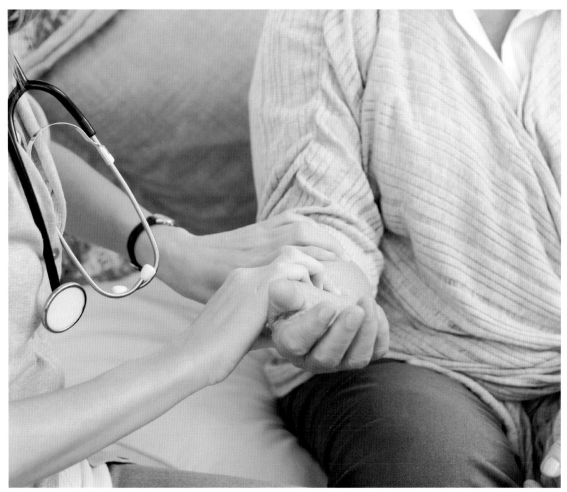

As we have emphasized throughout this book, the ongoing high blood sugar levels of diabetes can cause all sorts of damage throughout your body. That's why it's so important to get high blood sugar levels down into a healthy range and keep them there over the long haul. But in addition to your concerted efforts to get your blood sugar under control, there are additional steps you can take to help protect parts of your body that are especially vulnerable to injury and malfunction resulting from your diabetes, and prevent complications.

Your Eyes and Diabetes

The eyes are the windows to the soul, as the old saying goes. Some scientists estimate that when our vision is healthy, we get 70 to 80 percent of our information about the world through our eyes. We hold the gift of vision in such high regard that it has become a metaphor for wisdom and prescience. But when your eyesight goes on the blink (pardon the pun), metaphors aren't much help.

When you were diagnosed with diabetes, one of your first thoughts may have been: *Does this mean I'll go blind?* It's an understandable fear, since diabetes is the number one cause of blindness. Diabetic retinopathy, the result of damage to the retina caused by high glucose levels, is the leading form of eye disease among people with diabetes, affecting both type 1 and type 2 patients. And its toll has been increasing at an alarming rate. According to Prevent Blindness America and the National Eye Institute, the number of people age 40 and older living with diabetic retinopathy increased 89 percent between 2000 and 2012, to more than 7.5 million Americans. Diabetes increases the risk for other common eye diseases, too. And while aging results in natural changes to the eyes that can diminish vision—which is why reading glasses are a baby boomer fashion staple—diabetes can make matters worse.

How You See Life

Like so many body parts, the eyes customarily come in matching pairs. Each eye is roughly one inch in diameter, though only about one-sixth of it is visible; the rest of the orb is tucked into the eye socket. The portion of the eye seen by the outside world resembles a tiny fried egg. The white exterior is connective tissue called the sclera, while the colored center, actually a ring of tiny muscle fibers, is known as the iris. The iris contracts and dilates to alter the size of the pupil, a small, dark opening in the middle of the iris that controls how much light enters the eye.

The eye is frequently compared to a camera, with good reason. A thin, transparent shell called the cornea protects the outside of the eye and acts as a lens, focusing incoming light, which is directed to a second lens tucked behind the pupil. This interior lens changes shape to adjust the focus, then bounces light to the back of the eye, where a ring of nerve cells called the retina collects the light, converting it into electrical messages. These messages are then transferred along the optic nerve to the brain, which interprets the world that our eyes see.

Diabetic Retinopathy

In diabetic retinopathy, damage to the retina from high blood sugar interferes with the eye's ability to send information to the brain. It does not always cause symptoms. Some patients only know they have diabetic retinopathy because doctors discover evidence of the damage in an eye exam. However, the condition can lead to severe vision loss. In one study, 3.6 percent of patients with type 1 diabetes were legally blind, while about half as many type 2 patients had the same degree of vision loss. The National Eye Institute classifies four stages of diabetic retinopathy:

1. Mild nonproliferative retinopathy: The blood vessels in the retina may begin to swell and develop small bulges. Doctors call these bulges microaneurysms, because they resemble the blood vessel abnormalities that cause brain aneurysms. Blood vessels may leak blood or fluid, forming deposits called exudates.

2. Moderate nonproliferative retinopathy: Diabetes causes blockages in blood vessels throughout the body, and those within the eye are no exception. As retinopathy worsens, the tiny blood vessels that nourish the retina start to clog.

3. Severe nonproliferative retinopathy: At this stage, so many blood vessels in the retina become blocked that parts of the retina begin to starve. In a panic, the eye signals the brain to build new blood vessels to renourish the deprived parts.

4. Proliferative retinopathy: The brain triggers the growth of new blood vessels, a process called neovascularization. But the new vessels are weak and abnormal.

Nonproliferative retinopathy (sometimes called background retinopathy) may be very mild. However, as blood vessels begin to leak into the retina, vision may blur. Problems become more serious if leaky blood vessels cause the macula, an area of the retina, to swell, interfering with the ability to see fine details. When severe, this problem, called macular edema, can cause blindness. Vision may blur further as the capillaries, or small blood vessels, feeding the macula become blocked.

Proliferative retinopathy gets its name from the way new blood vessels proliferate, or grow rapidly, in the eyes to compensate for blocked or damaged blood vessels. Unfortunately, these frail replacement vessels do far more harm than good. They do a poor job of supplying blood, and these new vessels can break down and leak (or hemorrhage) into the vitreous, a gel-like substance in the center of the eye. A minor leak may result only in the appearance of a few "floaters" (spots that dance before your eyes). A major vitreous hemorrhage can cause significant vision loss and even blindness. The growth of new blood vessels can also produce scarring that may cause the retina to wrinkle or become detached, further damaging eyesight.

Other Eye Problems

Two other eye diseases that hit the diabetic population especially hard are glaucoma and cataracts.

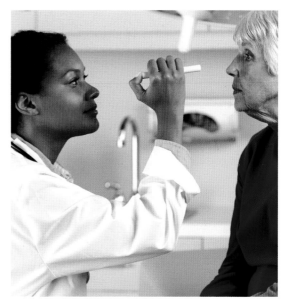

Glaucoma: This disease, which is estimated to afflict between two and three million Americans age 40 and older, is a leading cause of blindness in the United States. Glaucoma occurs when fluid fails to drain properly from the eyes, causing pressure to build and damage the optic nerve. There are several types of glaucoma. Diabetes raises the risk for neovascular glaucoma, a rare form of the disease. Diabetic retinopathy may cause the growth of new blood vessels on the iris, shutting off the flow of fluid and increasing pressure inside the eye. People with diabetes may be up to twice as likely to develop glaucoma as the general public.

Cataracts: More than 24 million Americans age 40 and older have cataracts, and half of Americans older than 80 have one or have had cataract surgery. Yet diabetes patients are still 60 percent more likely than others to develop this eye disorder. A cataract is a cloudiness caused by changes to fibers in the eye lens. Although a cataract may not cause complete blindness, it can block enough light to obscure visual details and clarity.

Seeing to Your Eyes

Maintaining tight control of your blood sugar can go a long way toward protecting your eyes. A study called the Diabetes Control and Complications Trial showed that aggressive insulin therapy dramatically reduces the risk of vision loss. In that study, researchers compared type 1 diabetes patients who gave themselves three or more insulin injections per day (or had an insulin pump) to another group of patients who received one or two insulin injections

daily. At the start of the study, none of the patients had signs of retinopathy. After an average of 6.5 years, patients in the aggressive-treatment group were 76 percent less likely to have developed retinopathy. (In an accompanying trial, patients who started with mild signs of retina damage cut in half their risk of further vision loss if they received aggressive insulin treatment.)

In addition, the following steps can help you preserve your sight.

Be on the lookout for trouble. Early signs that you may be developing diabetic retinopathy or another eye issue include:

- blurry or hazy vision
- "floaters" or spots that dance before your eyes
- night blindness
- increased sensitivity to glare, especially at night
- double vision
- loss of peripheral (side) vision
- difficulty reading
- a feeling of pressure in the eyes

If you notice any of these signs or any other changes in your vision, see your eye care professional as soon as possible. Don't dismiss vision problems as the effects of fatigue or aging, especially if they are persistent or seem to be getting worse. Early detection and intervention can often prevent problems from worsening and preserve remaining eyesight.

Have regular eye exams. Damage to the eye's blood supply that leads to vision loss can go on for years before symptoms arise, so regular examinations are critical. The American Diabetes Association recommends that all patients with type 1 disease undergo comprehensive screening for retinopathy within five years of being diagnosed with diabetes. Type 2 patients should have their eyes thoroughly examined soon after they are diagnosed with diabetes. After the initial screening, all diabetes patients should have an annual eye exam unless advised otherwise by their eye care professional. An optometrist or ophthalmologist should perform eye exams. If possible, find one who has experience in diagnosing and treating people with diabetes.

Lower your blood pressure. There are plenty of good reasons to keep blood pressure under control, such as lowering the risk for heart disease and stroke. However, high blood pressure also damages blood vessels in the retina, setting the stage for retinopathy. A large British study of more than 1,100 type 2 diabetes patients found that lowering high blood pressure reduced the risk of retinopathy by 34 percent over an eight-year period. Patients who maintained healthy blood pressure had sharper vision, too. (Not surprisingly, they also had fewer heart attacks and strokes.) So if you suffer from high blood pressure, be diligent about following your doctor's orders for treating it, including altering your diet, exercising regularly, tackling any weight problem, and taking medications as prescribed.

Don't smoke. And not just because all those clouds of smoke produced by puffing can obscure your vision. Tobacco users have a higher risk of diabetic retinopathy (and a

seemingly endless list of other serious medical problems). If you have diabetes and care a lick about your health (not to mention the well-being of those around you), you've got no business smoking or using any other form of tobacco.

Your Feet and Diabetes

Your feet are surprisingly complex structures. The two combined hold more than one-quarter of the bones in your body—26 each. And while they serve as a solid foundation, the feet aren't static blocks. Rather, they're agile and dynamic machines of movement, with more than 100 tendons, muscles, and ligaments apiece. Given all those moving parts and the pounding that the feet take every day, it's not surprising that, according to the American Podiatric Medical Association, about 75 percent of Americans experience one foot condition or another in their lifetime.

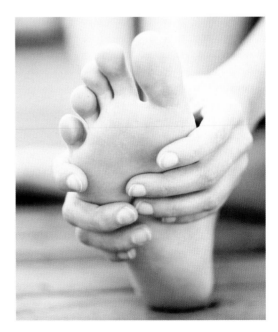

Add diabetes to the mix, however, and the pressure on the feet can become unbearable. Having the condition doubles a person's risk for foot disease. In fact, about 30 percent of people with diabetes who are older than 40 develop medical problems with their feet. And while blood sugar problems can create a dizzying range of hard-to-treat complications throughout the body, those that affect the lower legs and feet can progress with what seems like lightning speed. Indeed, in people with diabetes, lower-limb diseases that are not properly treated can deteriorate so quickly and so badly that doctors have no other choice but to remove the affected area in order to save their patients' lives. The sad result: People with diabetes account for more than 60 percent of all lower-limb amputations in the United States. A person with diabetes is 10 to 30 times more likely to have a lower limb amputated than is a person without the disease.

As you know all too well by now, the chronically elevated glucose levels of diabetes can damage the nervous system, the wiring that transmits signals from the brain throughout the body. The nervous system works the other way, too: It detects information about the environment and how it affects the body through the five senses. Damaged nerves, or neuropathy, can lead to an array of physical problems and disabilities anywhere in the body. But nerve injuries and other diseases that affect the feet and lower legs may be the complications most frequently associated with diabetes. What's more, the various foot conditions linked to diabetes may be the complications patients dread most.

Annoying and painful symptoms can occur when the brain can't successfully send messages to the feet. But the even greater threat posed by diabetic neuropathy happens when the feet can't send information to the brain because they've become numb from overexposure to blood sugar. Blisters, cuts, and other injuries that once would have made you wince or howl in pain go unnoticed when your feet lose their feeling.

To make matters worse, dulled nerves probably aren't your only problem if you have diabetes. The disease can also cause poor blood circulation. Like the heart's arteries, blood vessels elsewhere in the body can become stiff and narrowed. In fact, 1 in 3 diabetes sufferers over the age of 50 has clogged arteries in the legs, a condition known as peripheral artery disease or peripheral vascular disease. Narrowed arteries diminish blood flow to the lower legs and feet, which can cause pain during long-distance walks. More ominously, the loss of blood flow to the feet can prevent wounds and sores from getting the oxygen

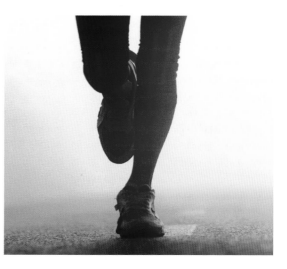

and nutrients required for healing, allowing these injuries to fester and spread.

So while occasional bumps, blisters, or cuts on the feet are trivial medical concerns for most people, for diabetes patients these minor injuries can turn serious in a hurry. Left unnoticed and untreated, minor sores on the skin of the foot can turn into severe problems with potentially devastating consequences—namely, foot ulcers.

Foot Ulcers

Most people think of ulcers as burning sores that cause bellyaches. But while gastric and peptic ulcers that form in the stomach and intestines are usually easy to cure with drugs, ulcers on the skin of the feet and legs can pose a more serious threat. These craterlike wounds can arise from seemingly inconsequential injuries to the feet. In extreme cases, they can deteriorate and develop into crippling complications.

According to the Centers for Disease Control and Prevention, about 15 percent of people with diabetes develop foot ulcers. The problems begin with nerve damage. Specifically, ulcers arise due to a loss of sensation in the foot caused by peripheral neuropathy. (About 60 to 70 percent of people with diabetes have some form of neuropathy.) If feeling in the lower limbs is lost, the risk of foot ulcers soars 700 percent.

When you lose sensation in the feet, small injuries can go unnoticed and degenerate into large, open sores. There are endless scenarios for how a foot ulcer may begin to form, including the following:

- If you have damaged nerves in the lower limbs, you may not be aware that a pair of ill-fitting shoes is causing blisters, corns, or other foot conditions that can lead to ulcers.

- If your skin can no longer distinguish hot from cold, you could scald your foot in steaming-hot bathwater; the burned skin may then blister.

- You could step on a sharp rock or bit of glass and cut your heel while walking barefoot.

- If your foot is numb from nerve damage, you may frequently bang it into hard objects without knowing it because you don't feel any pain. Over time, damage to joints and other structures in the foot could cause a deformity that puts pressure on the skin.

- If you have arthritis in the ankle or toes, you may lose joint mobility and alter the way you walk so that too much pressure is placed on the ball of the foot. Or, your normal gait may simply apply excessive force on certain sections of your soles. Over time, wear and tear could cause the skin to erode, forming a sore.

- Simply cutting your toenails the wrong way can damage skin and produce sores.

In addition to nerve damage, people with diabetes tend to have several other problems that further increase the risk of foot ulcers, such as:

- Poor blood flow. As mentioned, peripheral artery disease may reduce or cut off blood flow to the lower limbs, which will slow or prevent healing of sores (as well as make walking around the block a painful experience).

- Sugar-rich blood. Bacteria feast on glucose, so the combination of an open wound and high blood sugar can lead to raging infection.

- Decreased immune function. To make matters worse, diabetes interferes with the immune system's ability to kill germs, and that allows infections to worsen.

- Poor vision. If blood sugar has damaged your optic nerves, blurry vision can make detecting cuts and sores more difficult.

- Excess body fat. If you're overweight, as many type 2 diabetes patients are, simply bending over to examine or treat your feet may be difficult, if not impossible.

Foot ulcers and the complications they can cause are not an inevitable part of having diabetes, however. Along with maintaining healthy blood sugar, here are steps to keep these nasty sores at bay.

Meet your feet. Get to know them intimately. Make a point of examining your feet at least once a day. Be on the lookout for any cracks, cuts, sores, bumps, or bruises. Be sure to check between your toes. If necessary, use a hand mirror with a long handle or place a mirror on the floor to check areas that are hard to see. Report any problems to your doctor. If you have poor vision, ask someone else to give your feet a once-over.

Clean up your act. Washing your feet daily will do more than keep them from smelling like, well, feet. Good foot hygiene can help prevent infections. To avoid burns, be sure to test water temperature with your hand before stepping into a bath or—better yet—use a thermometer; 90 to 95 degrees Fahrenheit should be about right. Use mild, nonabrasive, unscented soap that contains lanolin, a moisturizer. Dry each foot carefully with a clean towel, especially between the toes. Most doctors discourage patients with foot ulcers from soaking their feet for too long because it robs the skin of its natural protective oils and, ironically, can actually result in dry skin.

Wear sensible shoes. "These shoes are killing me!" is the familiar refrain from sore-footed sorts after a day of wearing too-tight pumps or wingtips. While uncomfortable shoes may not be deadly weapons, they can cause foot problems that may turn serious if left untreated. One study of 669 patients with foot ulcers found that about 20 percent of the sores were linked to ill-fitting footwear that caused rubbing on the skin.

Get hosed. Wearing stockings or socks will help prevent foot problems. Opt for those that help your feet stay dry. Stay away from tight socks or hose, which can reduce circulation. Check that any seams are not bunched up between your toes and inside of the shoe, which can cause blisters. No matter what type of socks or hose you wear, change them once a day (or more often if your feet sweat a lot).

Don't go barefoot in the park. Or in the backyard, or on the beach, or anywhere else, for that matter, including inside your own home. Hot pavement or sand can burn your feet, sharp pebbles or shards of glass can cause gashes, and you can accidentally stub your toe or kick a hard object just about anywhere. When you're at the beach, lake, or ocean, wear beach or water shoes, which offer more protection than flip-flops. (Wear them at public locker rooms and pools, too, to protect against viruses and fungi.) Find a sturdy pair of slippers to wear around the house.

Get 'em checked regularly. Plan to have a thorough foot exam at least once a year, more often if you smoke or have any other condition that raises the risk of ulcers and complications. If you have been diagnosed with neuropathy, ask your physician to have a look at your feet every chance you get. As a reminder for both you and your doctor, take your shoes and socks off as soon as you're shown to the exam table.

Your Skin and Diabetes

If you are tempted to flip past this section because you think skin care is for sissies, think again, buster. Skin damage is a major complication of diabetes, with the potential to produce everything from barely noticeable blemishes to disfiguring scars. What's more, maintaining healthy skin is crucial for warding off disease and protecting your innards from the perils of the outside world.

As a matter of fact, every diabetes patient should get to know his or her skin better. By examining yourself every day, from head to toe, you may be able to spot small problems before they turn into serious ones. And, as you'll learn, the skin problems described in the following pages can serve as a caution that greater health concerns may lie beneath the surface.

Diabetes patients do not have a monopoly on skin problems, of course. Walk into any pharmacy or supermarket and you will find aisles overflowing with emollients, creams, astringents, and salves—evidence that damaged skin is a consuming cosmetic and medical concern for the general population. However, having diabetes appears to increase the risk for rashes, sores, and other conditions.

According to the American Diabetes Association, about one-third of patients will develop a skin disorder at some point. And as you just learned, the skin on your lower extremities is particularly vulnerable to problems.

The Skin You're In

As every child learns in school, the skin is the largest organ in the body. Your hide has a surface area of about two square yards and weighs about 10 pounds. Your skin acts as a protective covering for your bones, muscles, and organs. However, the skin is more than mere armor, with many of its critical roles performed below the exterior.

The body's outer shell, called the epidermis, is made up of a top layer of skin cells that are dead. That's just as well, since they are constantly flaking and peeling off anyway. Fortunately, the body replaces these so-called horny cells just as quickly with new ones, as cells in the lower layer of the epidermis divide. Some cells in the epidermis produce melanin, the pigment that provides skin color.

Beneath the epidermis lies the dermis. Hidden from sight, this layer is packed with vital equipment that keeps the skin healthy and performs various functions. In the health-and-beauty department, there are hair follicles and sebaceous glands, which produce oil called sebum that moistens the skin. The dermis also contains nerve endings, which detect pain and pressure and govern the sense of touch. They also sense temperature, advising the brain when it's time to slip on a sweater or change into shorts. Furthermore, the dermis is home to sweat glands, which help regulate body temperature by producing cooling perspiration. Blood vessels constrict to conserve body heat when you're cold, along with their usual duties of providing nourishment to all of the skin and its various structures.

The third and innermost tier of the skin is called the subcutaneous layer. Mostly made up of fat, it provides insulation and protects bones and organs from bumps and bangs.

How Diabetes Affects Your Skin

High blood sugar can rough up smooth skin in several ways. Elevated glucose results in high levels of compounds called advanced glycosylation end products (AGEs), which damage nerves and blood vessels that are necessary to keep skin healthy. However, your body's defense against high blood sugar may cause collateral damage to the epidermis, as you'll read in a moment. The first two major conditions we'll discuss, dry skin and skin infections, are common medical problems that can affect anyone, whether they have diabetes or not. However, people who have the disease are far more likely to develop these skin conditions. Many of the lesser-known skin problems discussed later primarily afflict people with diabetes.

Dry Skin

If you spend all day scratching and your skin would make an iguana blush, chances are you're going to flunk your next blood-sugar test. When glucose levels rise too high, the body tries to get rid of the excess sugar through frequent urination. The more you urinate, the more fluid your body loses. If you don't replace that lost fluid by guzzling lots of water, you become dehydrated, which causes (among other symptoms) dry skin.

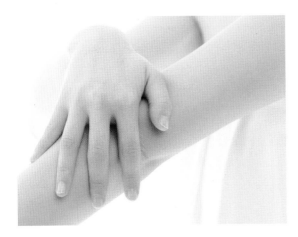

As skin loses moisture, it becomes itchy. In severe cases, red scales may form. Scratching can cause sores to crack, opening the skin to an invasion of infectious bacteria. Damage to blood vessels and nerve endings in the skin from high glucose levels makes matters worse.

Of course, you don't need diabetes to develop dry skin. But people with diabetes need to be particularly wary of the environmental influences that can turn anyone's skin to parchment. In cold climates, winter is a worrisome time, since heating systems sap the air of indoor humidity and cold winds chap the skin. Hot showers or baths with soaps and shampoos strip protective sebum from the skin any time of year.

To prevent dry skin, follow these steps:

Shorten your showers. Long, hot showers or baths may feel great, but they strip away natural oil that keeps skin soft and moist. Bathe in warm water, use mild soap and shampoo, and don't linger too long. Pat yourself dry with a towel.

Stay well lubed. Apply skin moisturizer after you bathe. Ask your doctor to recommend a brand. Slather the stuff on liberally everywhere except between the toes, which should be kept dry to avoid the fungal infections.

Drink up. Water, that is, to keep your body well hydrated.

Get misty. Unless you live in a tropical climate, use a humidifier to keep the air in your home and workplace from becoming dry during cold winter months.

Skin Infections

Skin infections can afflict anyone, too, but doctors agree that having diabetes greatly increases the risk for an invasion of microscopic meanies. The bacteria called *Staphylococcus aureus* (better known as staph) and the fungus *Candida albicans* cause many of the skin infections that are most common among people with diabetes.

Some of the more common bacterial skin infections to watch out for include these:

Boils. (Warning: The following definition gets pretty icky, fast.) Boils are painful red lumps that usually occur when bacteria infect a hair follicle. As inflammation worsens, the boil fills with pus and forms a yellow head before rupturing and draining. (Told you so.) Any part of the skin can develop a boil, although these ghastly little sores seem to like hairy areas, for obvious reasons, especially where you sweat a lot. (That means that the face, neck, armpits, and other sweat-inducing zones are most likely to get "boiled.") Hot compresses may relieve pain and make a boil heal faster. If a painful boil persists, see a doctor, who may drain the sore and give you a prescription for antibiotics. Above all, don't squeeze or pop a boil, which could worsen an infection.

Carbuncles. When a bunch of boils gang together, they form a carbuncle. Because they are more serious than single boils, you should see a doctor.

Sties. A sty is like a boil, only it forms on the edge of or under the eyelid. A sty may be painful or grow large enough to block vision. Warm compresses may relieve pain and encourage a sty to shrink, but see a doctor if the problem persists. Antibiotic creams can help heal a sty and prevent recurrence. Never squeeze or pierce a sty.

Some of the more common fungal infections (also known as tinea corporis) to afflict people with diabetes include these related conditions:

Athlete's foot. You don't have to be a jock to get this itchy, scaly menace.

Jock itch. Likewise, you don't have to wear an athletic supporter to develop this uncomfortable condition, though those snug-fitting protective garments can contribute to the problem (which explains why jock itch usually afflicts males). Also known as tinea cruris, the problem begins as an itchy red rash around the genitals, which can spread to the inner thigh.

Ringworm. As the name suggests, this fungal infection forms ring-shape scales on the skin that may itch. (Fortunately, it doesn't mean you have worms, though having an infectious fungus is nothing to brag about.) Ringworm often develops on the scalp, though it can turn up on other parts of the body. Ringworm of the toenails and fingernails, called onychomycosis, is a common problem. The nails turn thick and discolored, and there's not much your manicurist can do about it.

Fungal infections can turn up on other parts of the body, too. Over-the-counter medications may help, but your physician can prescribe a more powerful antifungal drug to clear up persistent problems.

To prevent skin infections:

Keep it clean. We know, we know, we just got done telling you that bathing too often can worsen dry skin. But that doesn't mean you should avoid bathing. A thorough daily cleaning will keep bacteria at bay.

Keep it dry. Again, isn't dry skin a threat? Yes, but so are dark, damp places on the body, such as between the toes and under the arms, where fungus can grow. Using a little talcum powder on areas where skin rubs against skin isn't a bad idea.

APPENDIX A: CARB EXCHANGE LIST

1 vegetable exchange

(5 grams carbohydrate) equals:

½ **cup** Vegetables, cooked (carrots, broccoli, zucchini, cabbage, etc.)

1 **cup** Vegetables, raw, or salad greens

½ **cup** Vegetable juice

1 milk exchange

(12 grams carbohydrate) equals:

1 **cup** Milk: fat-free, 1% fat, 2%, or whole

¾ **cup** Yogurt, plain nonfat or low-fat

1 **cup** Yogurt, artificially sweetened

1 fruit exchange

(15 grams carbohydrate) equals:

1 **small** Apple, banana, orange, or nectarine

1 **medium** Peach

1 **whole** Kiwi

½ Grapefruit or mango

1 **cup** Berries, fresh (strawberries, rasp berries, blueberries)

1 **cup** Melon, fresh, cubes

1 **slice** Melon, honeydew or cantaloupe

½ **cup** Juice (orange, apple, or grape)

4 **teaspoons** Jelly or jam

1 starch exchange

(15 grams carbohydrate) equals:

1 **slice** Bread (white, pumpernickel, whole-wheat, rye)

2 **slices** Bread, reduced-calorie or "lite"

¼ **(1 oz)** Bagel, bakery-style

½ Bagel, frozen, or English muffin

½ Bun, hamburger or hot dog

1 **small** Dinner roll

¾ **cup** Cold cereal

⅓ **cup** Rice (cooked), brown or white

⅓ **cup** Barley or couscous, cooked

⅓ **cup** Legumes (dried beans, peas, lentils)

½ **cup** Beans, cooked (black or kidney beans, chick peas)

½ **cup** Pasta, cooked

½ **cup** Corn, potato, or green peas

3 **ounces** Potato, baked, sweet or white

¾ **ounce** Pretzels

3 **cups** Popcorn, air-popped or microwaved

APPENDIX A: CARB EXCHANGE LIST

1 meat exchange

(0 grams carbohydrate) equals:

1 ounce	Beef, pork, turkey, or chicken
1 ounce	Fish fillet (flounder, sole, scrod, cod, etc.)
1 ounce	Tuna or sardines, canned
1 ounce	Shellfish (clams, lobster, scallops, shrimp)
¾ cup	Cottage cheese, nonfat or low-fat
1 ounce	Cheese, shredded or sliced
1 ounce	Lunch meat
1 whole	Egg
¼ cup	Egg substitute
4 ounces	Tofu

1 fat exchange

(0 grams carbohydrate) equals:

1 teaspoon	Oil (vegetable, corn, canola, olive, etc.)
1 teaspoon	Butter
1 teaspoon	Margarine, stick
1 teaspoon	Mayonnaise
1 Tablespoon	Margarine or mayonnaise, reduced-fat
1 Tablespoon	Salad dressing
1 Tablespoon	Cream cheese
2 Tablespoons	Lite cream cheese
1/8	Avocado
8 large	Black olives
10 large	Green olives, stuffed
1 slice	Bacon

APPENDIX B: GLYCEMIC INDEX OF COMMON FOODS

Bread/Crackers

Bagel...................................72
Graham crackers........................ 74
Hamburger bun............................61
Kaiser roll..............................73
Pita bread...............................57
Pumpernickel bread......................51
Rye bread, dark..........................76
Rye bread, light.........................55
Saltines................................ 74
Sourdough bread......................... 52
Wheat bread, high-fiber.................68
White bread..............................71

Cakes/Cookies/Muffins

Angel food cake..........................67
Banana bread.............................47
Blueberry muffin........................ 59
Chocolate cake.......................... 38
Corn muffin.............................102
Cupcake with icing......................73
Donut...................................76
Oat bran muffin..........................60
Oatmeal cookie..........................55
Pound cake..............................54
Shortbread cookies...................... 64

Candy

Jelly beans............................. 80
Lifesavers..............................70
M&M's, peanut...........................33
Milky Way Bar...........................44

Cereals/Breakfast

All-Bran................................42

Bran flakes

Bran flakes............................. 74
Cheerios............................... 74
Cocoa Krispies..........................77
Corn flakes.............................83
Cream of wheat......................... 70
Frosted Flakes......................... 55
Golden Grahams......................... 71
Grape Nuts.............................67
Life...................................66
Oatmeal................................ 49
Pancakes...............................67
Puffed Wheat...........................67
Raisin Bran............................ 73
Rice Bran.............................. 19
Rice Krispies.......................... 82
Shredded Wheat......................... 69
Special K.............................. 66
Total..................................76
Waffles................................76

Dairy

Chocolate milk.........................34
Ice cream, vanilla.....................62
Ice cream, chocolate...................68
Milk, skim............................ 32
Milk, whole............................27
Soy milk.............................. 30
Yogurt, low-fat........................33

Fruits/Juices

Apple.................................. 38
Apple juice............................ 41
Apricot................................57
Banana.................................55
Cantaloupe.............................65

191

Cherries... 22	
Cranberry juice....................................... 68	
Dates... 103	
Fruit cocktail... 55	
Grapefruit... 25	
Grapefruit juice....................................... 48	
Grapes... 46	
Orange... 44	
Orange juice... 52	
Peach.. 42	
Pear.. 37	
Pineapple... 66	
Pineapple juice.. 46	
Plum.. 39	
Raisins... 64	
Watermelon... 72	

Rice/Grains

Brown rice.. 55
Couscous.. 65
Instant rice... 87
Long-grain rice.. 56
Risotto... 69
Vermicelli... 58

Snack Foods

Corn chips.. 74
Granola bar... 61
Peanuts.. 15
Popcorn.. 55
Potato chips.. 54
Pretzels.. 81
Rice cakes.. 77

Legumes

Baked beans.. 48
Black beans... 30
Black-eyed peas....................................... 42
Chick peas.. 33
Fava beans.. 79
Lentils, red... 25
Lima beans.. 32
Peas, dried... 22
Pinto beans... 45
Red kidney beans...................................... 19

Soups

Black bean.. 64
Lentil... 44
Minestrone.. 39
Split pea.. 60
Tomato... 38

Sugars/Spreads

Honey.. 58
Strawberry jam.. 51

Pasta

Fettuccini... 32
Gnocchi.. 68
Linguini.. 55
Macaroni.. 45
Macaroni and cheese................................. 64
Ravioli with meat...................................... 39
Spaghetti.. 41
Spaghetti, wheat...................................... 37

Vegetables

French fries.. 75
Potato, baked.. 85
Potato, mashed.. 91
Carrots, boiled... 49
Carrots, raw.. 16
Carrots, sweet... 55
Peas.. 48
Sweet potato... 44